PRACTITIONER RESEARCH

FOR SOCIAL WORK, NURSING, AND THE HEALTH PROFESSIONS

PRACTITIONER RESEARCH

FOR SOCIAL WORK, NURSING, AND THE HEALTH PROFESSIONS

Payam Sheikhattari

Michael T. Wright

Gillian B. Silver

Cyrilla van der Donk

Bas van Lanen

JOHNS HOPKINS UNIVERSITY PRESS

Baltimore

This book is an adaptation of a Dutch work titled *Praktijkonderzoek in zorg en welzijn*, authored by Cyrilla van der Donk and Bas van Lanen and originally published in 2011 by Uitgeverij Coutinho.

English translation of the original Dutch work by Manon Massizzo.

Dr. Anne Marie O'Keefe prepared the index for this edition.

Johns Hopkins University Press
2715 North Charles Street
Baltimore, Maryland 21218–4363
www.press.jhu.edu

Library of Congress Cataloging-in-Publication Data

Names: Sheikhattari, Payam, 1971– author. | Wright, Michael T., author. | Silver, Gillian, author. | van der Donk, Cyrilla, 1961– author. | van Lanen, Bas, 1977– author.

Title: Practitioner research for social work, nursing, and the health professions / Payam Sheikhattari, Michael T. Wright, Gillian B. Silver, Cyrilla van der Donk, Bas van Lanen.

Description: Baltimore : Johns Hopkins University Press, [2022] | Includes bibliographical references and index.

Identifiers: LCCN 2020057358 | ISBN 9781421442051 (paperback ; alk. paper) | ISBN 9781421442068 (ebook)

Subjects: MESH: Health Services Research—methods | Nursing Research—methods | Research Design

Classification: LCC RA409 | NLM W 84.3 | DDC 362.1072/3—dc23

LC record available at https://lccn.loc.gov/2020057358

A catalog record for this book is available from the British Library.

Special discounts are available for bulk purchases of this book. For more information, please contact Special Sales at specialsales@jh.edu.

Contents

Preface

Practitioner research is an important investment for both individual practitioners and the organizations in which they serve. Research can be used for evaluation, quality improvement, and solving practice problems, and the approach can empower professionals to generate support, enhance their professional knowledge and skills, improve their self-confidence, and advance their collective ability in changing a situation.

This book provides step-by-step instructions for conducting practitioner research in social work, nursing, and other professional settings in health care and social welfare. Our goal is to introduce an easy-to-navigate process through which practitioners gradually become more competent in collecting and using research data (figure P.1).

After a thorough introduction to practitioner research and its core principles (chapter 1), each of the following chapters describes one of the seven key components of the Practitioner Research Method, including real examples and exercises from professional practice. In each stage, the steps are described in detail, along with specific techniques and methods for implementing the steps. This book can be used as a guide for both seasoned professionals as well as students just starting to engage in their own research.

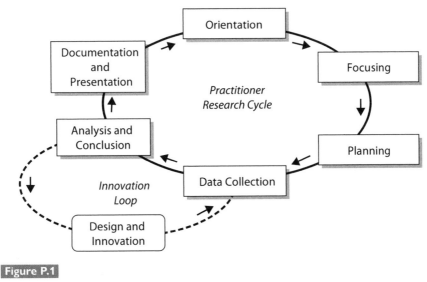

Figure P.1

Practitioner Research Method

Chapter 1 compares and positions practitioner research in relation to other forms of systematic inquiries. First, specific details are provided on the rationale for conducting practitioner research, the expected outcomes, historical roots, and underlying philosophy. Second, the benefits of practitioner research are discussed and explored, followed by an overview of the Practitioner Research Method's key components. Later, the chapter summarizes the methodological principles of practitioner research along with practical implementation strategies and examples of various types of research questions and designs. At the end, general considerations for conducting practitioner research in health care and social service settings are examined.

Chapter 2 is dedicated to topics related to orientation, the first key component of the Practitioner Research Method. These include common reasons that some practitioners become interested in engaging in research, several techniques that can help a practitioner identify and select a significant practice problem, and explorative methods that can lead to a more in-depth understanding of an issue from multiple perspectives. The information gained through this first step is used to further define the practice problem in a way that could be used to determine the "focus" of the practitioner research, the next key component of the cycle.

Chapter 3 systematically guides practitioners through effectively focusing their research by providing technical instructions for performing an in-depth problem analysis. The results of the analysis help formulate research objectives, which will guide the process of identifying and formulating important research questions and their respective sub-questions.

Chapter 4 introduces relevant data collection tools that can be developed and used in the planning stage of practitioner research. First, questions are introduced that can help identify methods for data collection. Next, methods for identifying target groups and estimating the number of needed respondents are described. Lastly, various tools and guidelines for preparing an effective work plan, as well as standardizing and assessing the cohesiveness of a research plan, are discussed.

Chapter 5 is a deep dive into data collection and provides specific details on practical data collection tools and activities that can be used in professional practice settings. First, data collection instruments are discussed followed by further exploration of the main data collection methods of practitioner research: document analysis, systematic observation, interviewing, surveying, testing, alternative data collection methods, and site visits.

Chapter 6 describes the key component of "analysis and conclusion," the stage during which the answers to research questions are extracted from the collected data. Every step of this component, from preparing collected data for analysis to drawing conclusions, is specified and discussed. First, different types of data (qualitative, quantitative) are described, followed by introducing specific methods used for analyzing them. Second, useful approaches for formulating conclusions from the analyzed data are explained. Lastly, general recommendations for strengthening the analysis and conclusion process are provided.

Chapter 7 provides specific information related to practitioner research studies with the objective of solving a practice problem by developing and testing a new intervention. Two phases of design research are described. The first phase consists of exploratory research to collect and analyze data needed for identifying the key elements (design principles) for a possible intervention. The second phase is called the Innovation Loop, which guides the development and implementation of the intervention. In this chapter, the steps taken in the first phase of design research are described, focusing on the design principles, followed by describing the design and innovation that occurs during the Innovation Loop. Lastly, the method of rapid prototyping is addressed.

Chapter 8 presents the concepts of dissemination and implementation of research results, formally called "documentation and presentation." This includes the importance of considering the characteristics and interests of the target audience, various communication strategies for disseminating the findings (mainly in the form of a report and/or other types of presentations), the concept of implementing innovative activities informed by the findings, followed by strategies that could maximize their impact. Lastly, we explore topics such as evaluation of the research, reflection, and future recommendations.

As a final service to our readers and fellow research practitioners, we have provided an appendix that summarizes different sources, and strategies for identifying the most appropriate ones, as well as how to assess and reference sources throughout the research cycle. The appendix can be referred to at any time in the research process.

PRACTITIONER RESEARCH

FOR SOCIAL WORK, NURSING, AND THE HEALTH PROFESSIONS

1

An Introduction to Practitioner Research

The idea of involving service providers in research is not new. Throughout history, several of the most prominent contributors to health and social sciences have been men and women who were at home in both the worlds of practice and academia. For example, Sigmund Freud conducted most of the preliminary research leading to his psychoanalysis theory based on assessing his own unconscious impulses as well as observing and interviewing his patients (BBC History, 2014). With the explosion of new discoveries, the exponential increase in the amount of knowledge being produced, and the growing demands of practice, both the production and application of knowledge have become highly specialized and increasingly complex, which has resulted in a widening gap between research and practice. Practitioner research is a way to close that gap.

In this chapter, we first compare practitioner research to other forms of scientific investigation and ways of knowing and then discuss the specific rationale that practitioners bring to the table as well as the expected outcomes, historical roots, and underlying philosophy of practitioner research. We also consider the benefits of conducting practitioner research both for practitioners and their organizations, and we introduce the key components of the Practitioner Research Method, each followed by an illustrative example from the field. The methodological principles of practitioner research (such as validity and reliability) are presented, along with an exploration of practical strategies for their implementation and the various types of practitioner research questions and their respective designs. Lastly, we examine general considerations for conducting practitioner research in health care and social service settings. At the end of this chapter, we provide a brief summary and exercises.

1.1. Positioning Practitioner Research

Practitioner Research Defined

The goal of practitioner research is to study professional practice within its local context for the purpose of generating knowledge on how to improve services. It empowers service providers to collect and analyze data as an active part of professional practice, conducted as an integrated part of health care and social service delivery. Improving professional practice doesn't necessarily mean that you always have to make changes by implementing new interventions and designs, however. Simply gaining a better understanding of how the professional practice functions is seen as an improvement in practitioner research.

Definition of Practitioner Research

Practitioner research consists of empirical studies conducted by social workers, nurses, and other health professionals to answer questions resulting from their practices. The research takes place as an interaction between the practitioner doing the research and his or her colleagues, patients, or clients. The primary goal of practitioner research is to improve one's own practice.

Practitioner research as defined here draws from traditions in the United Kingdom, Australia, and the Netherlands originating in the field of education (teacher research) and expanding to health care and social welfare professionals in more recent years. These traditions are based in action research, design research, and participatory health research approaches. Practitioner research in relation to these traditions is defined in table 1.1.

Table 1.1. Practitioner research and related research traditions		
Research tradition	Definition	Relation to practitioner research
Action research	"Action research seeks to bring together action and reflection, theory and practice, in participation with others, in the pursuit of practical solutions to issues of pressing concern to people, and more generally the flourishing of individual persons and their communities" (Reason & Bradbury, 2001, p. 1)	Practitioner research shares many elements with action research, such as the involvement of internal stakeholders in research and its practical approach to generate actions and practical solutions to the pressing issues. What differentiates practitioner research from action research is its methodological approach according to a framework adapted for professional practice settings.
Design research	Researchers design and test interventions that solve practical problems in order to generate effective interventions and theory useful for guiding design and changing the status quo (Van den Akker, 1999)	Design research follows a cycle of designing, evaluating, and revising. It aims to improve professional practice, but it is not necessarily conducted by the practitioners themselves. Practitioner research is specific to professional practice and is conducted by the practitioners.
Participatory health research	Participatory health research is an orientation to research—not a methodological approach—to maximize the participation of those whose life or work is the subject of the research in all stages of the research process (ICPHR, 2013)	Practitioner research in the health care field is a form of participatory health research conducted under the leadership of practitioners in collaboration with their clients/patients and others in every stage of the process. Practitioner research is described as a set of specific methods relevant to practice settings.

The Importance of an Inquisitive Mind-Set

Van Vliet (2009) draws attention to the importance of an inquisitive mind-set as the starting point for practitioner research. This is characterized by critical thinking and reflection on one's practice by asking new questions about why a particular phenomenon exists, how it can change, who can make the change, and what resources are needed. Answers to these questions can lead to a deeper understanding and a higher motivation for change. Through an inquisitive mind-set, one can gain in-depth knowledge of the issues and develop interesting, innovative ideas that could inspire others and provide the necessary support for conducting research. Sharing knowledge with colleagues and clients/patients creates further opportunities for reflection through dialogue. Professional reflection requires active listening and being open to learning from other perspectives, which are important skills to practice. These skills enable you to step back and consider your thoughts and experiences in relation to those coming from your environment (e.g., your clients/patients, organization, or professional society). Methods to foster an inquisitive mind-set include keeping a journal for documentation and reflection, being a mentee, or mentoring others. This book provides ample opportunities for practicing critical thinking and reflection throughout the process of designing and conducting practitioner research.

The Added Value of Practitioner Research

Knowledge and expertise in practice settings can quickly become outdated. Learning on the part of professionals in the interest of improving their practice requires asking questions, making intentional observations, and sharing ideas and knowledge. The internet, the published literature, continuing education, and conversations with other experts are important. However, increasing demands, limited resources, and time constraints often leave practitioners with little time for such activities. Further, these sources often do not address directly the questions that practitioners face in their everyday practices, which include novel situations and difficult and recurring problems specific to their setting. That's why practitioners cannot solely rely on the usual learning opportunities for staying up to date and providing the best possible care. A systematic, empirical approach embedded in daily work routines provides new insights that in turn serve as a basis for innovation in practice. Practitioner research enables practitioners to learn systematically from their own experience. In addition, practitioner research studies have the potential to save time and costs, the savings being the result of improved practice, an enhanced capacity for problem-solving, and a broadened understanding of the bigger picture and the real needs of clients/patients.

Van Keken (2006) defines three levels of professional competency:

- Level I: *Professional services competencies* defined as the necessary skills and expertise related to the provision of services such as counseling, treatment, and therapies.
- Level II: *Professional environment competencies* related to the functioning of practitioners in their own organizations and in collaboration with colleagues and management.

- Level III: *Professional practice competencies* related to career advancement and contributions to their fields of professional practice (e.g., new concepts and models for practice).

The methods and techniques described in this book are intended to help practitioners enhance and maintain all three levels.

Practitioner Research, Evidence-Based Practice, and Other Forms of Research

Despite considerable investment in health and social research, little attention has been paid to ensuring that research findings inform and improve practice (Bero et al., 1998; Smith & Wilkins, 2018). It has been shown in the health care field that "it takes an average of 17 years for research evidence to reach clinical practice" (Balas & Boren, 2000, p. 66). There is no shortage of academic research, but not all successful studies find their way fast enough into the development of innovative solutions. Expediting the process of moving from discovery to implementation will bring our collective investment in research to fruition (Brownson, 2017). But first we need to understand what stands in the way of translating research knowledge into practice.

The primary problem is the divide that exists between the academic researchers who are expected to produce new knowledge and the practitioners who are regarded as the consumers of that knowledge. In the medical field this divide goes by many names: for example, *bench to bedside*, *basic to applied*, or *diffusion of innovation* (Brownson, 2017; Rogers & Shoemaker, 1971). In 2003, the National Institutes of Health (NIH) in the United States published the *NIH Roadmap*, which explicitly names the need to "translate" basic and clinical research more quickly into clinical and community-based practices (Zerhouni, 2003). The *NIH Roadmap* defines four stages (T1–T4): T1 is the translation of basic science (nonhuman subjects) into clinical research concepts (human subjects); T2 encompasses the three phases of clinical trials to test the efficacy of the treatments in human subjects; T3 is dissemination and implementation of the research to market the new treatment and innovations into health practices; and finally, T4 is focused on the evaluation of real-world outcomes and the effectiveness of the adapted versions of the research in diverse contexts (Brownson, 2017; Westfall et al., 2007; Zerhouni, 2003).

The knowledge gap between research and practice has also been discussed in terms of *evidence-based practice* (EBP): practice should be based on interventions that have proven to be effective under scientific conditions. EBP is defined as the conscientious, explicit, and judicious use of current best *evidence* (that is, the results from research studies) in making decisions about the care provided to patients or clients. EBP originated in medicine, based on the empirical observation that what practitioners believe to be the best care is too often not based on what research has shown to work (Sackett, 1997). The concept of EBP has since been carried over to other health care and social welfare professions. EBP is often misunderstood as being a direct application of research findings to practice. However, it actually promotes the integration of the best available evidence from all academic studies to date (in the form of systematic reviews), the practitioner's experience and judgement, and the concerns of the client/patient

(Sackett, 1997). A central critique of the EBP concept is that academic research is conducted under highly controlled conditions that do not resemble the real world of practice (Westfall et al., 2007). Such studies can thus show that something works under those conditions, but it proves not to be effective in the practice setting. In other words, most of what is considered evidence in terms of EBP is not practice-based and therefore not practicable (Green, 2006).

Recognizing this critique, the concept of EBP has been expanded in more recent years to include not just studies showing the efficacy of interventions under controlled conditions, but also how the evidence from such studies is implemented by practitioners and with what effect. The focus on implementation requires more flexible research designs and both qualitative and quantitative methods of data collection and interpretation, incorporating participatory and systems sciences approaches (Green, 2006). This enables us to generate a new kind of evidence: *practice-based evidence* (PBE), which has a greater validity from a practitioner point of view and thus a greater potential for dissemination across diverse settings and participants. This new approach is often referred to as *implementation science* or *implementation research*: the study of integrating evidence-based interventions into a practice setting (Brownson, 2017). Implementation science aims at increasing the usefulness, feasibility, and scalability of new scientific evidence. Such research studies need to be conducted in diverse settings by those who directly provide services to patients and clients from different backgrounds.

Practitioner research can be seen as a particular form of implementation science in which empirical studies are conducted by practitioners themselves to answer questions resulting from their practice. Such studies do not just examine how knowledge generated by academic institutions can be applied in practice, but they also generate new knowledge in their own right. Research takes place where services are delivered and is integrated into routine interactions between the practitioner researcher and their colleagues and clients/patients. Hence, the primary goal of practitioner research is to improve the impact of practitioners in a specific setting by enhancing the quality and effectiveness of their services. It can also be defined as an empirically based strategic approach for organizational development in a real-life practice environment (Bolhuis, 2012; Harinck, 2007; Maykus, 2010; Van der Donk & Van Lanen, 2019; Van der Donk & Van Lanen, 2020; Van der Donk et al., 2014). The methods and techniques described in this book are intended to make it easier for practitioners to design and conduct valid research studies in their practice, taking into account the realistic opportunities available for organizational change.

This quality of practitioner research also distinguishes it from other forms of research common in the health care and social welfare fields that are focused on producing generalizable theoretical frameworks and models: namely, *basic research* and *intervention research*. Basic research in the social welfare and health care fields seeks to identify and understand the mechanisms underlying health and social problems at the individual, organizational, and societal levels. The findings provide a foundation for practitioners, policy makers, and others responding to emerging needs by informing them about the factors causing the problems. Intervention research focuses on ways to address the causes of the problems by developing and evaluating possible solutions. The solutions are in the form of interventions at any level of the problem, from the individual treatment of affected persons, to population-based campaigns, to improvements in service delivery systems, to new public policies at the local, regional, national, or international levels. Practitioner research complements basic research and intervention research by taking into account the findings of both while providing new knowledge to answer questions posed in a specific setting. For an overview of the relationship between these three types of research, see table 1.2.

Epistemologically, practitioner research is founded on a constructivist understanding of science, a characteristic of both action research and participatory health research. According to a constructivist approach, learning is an active process of constructing knowledge rather than acquiring it. Therefore, multiple versions of reality can exist and these are created based on the experiences and characteristics of the learners (Cooper, 1993). Much of academic research is based on the positivist approach instead, particularly as found in quantitative study designs. The positivist approach assumes that there is one reality to a social phenomenon that is discovered through scientific inquiry. Positivist study designs depend on inferential statistics, hypothesis testing, and reproducible methods with the purpose of uncovering "the underlying reality unknown to us" in a controlled environment (Lee, 1991). The positivist approach, with its emphasis on methodological precision and the standardization of research metrics, has resulted in important scientific discoveries and innovations, particularly in the natural sciences. However, this approach faces major limitations when exploring social phenomena, particularly when the research is focused on emergent knowledge in a specific context. The positivist approach requires highly controlled environments to minimize different biases and confounding effects. Such quantitative studies often use strict inclusion and exclusion criteria, detailed and standardized research protocols, randomization of the human subjects into cases and controls, and so on. These conditions cannot be met within everyday practice settings. The focus of such studies is also not the production of context-specific knowledge but rather generalizable results.

Table 1.2. A comparison of basic research, intervention research, and practitioner research			
	Basic research	Intervention research	Practitioner research
Purpose	Creating generalizable knowledge on the causes of health and social problems	Developing and evaluating solutions to health and social problems	Improving professional practices and enhancing organizational capacity to address health and social problems in a specific setting
Example 1	A national study to assess the burden of post-traumatic stress disorder (PTSD) and associated factors among war veterans	A study to assess the Veteran Affairs (VA) PTSD treatment and reimbursement policy and procedures	A study to improve health care provided to patients who suffer from PTSD in a specific VA clinic
Example 2	A study examining the association between the use of electronic cigarettes and poor health outcomes among high school students in Baltimore City, Maryland	A study to assess the quality and scope of tobacco control education, counseling, and social services provided in Baltimore City high schools	A study exploring the possibility of using youth peer advocates to educate Baltimore City high school regular e-cig users and to refer them to treatment

Practitioner research makes use of both qualitative and quantitative methods of data collection; however, the underlying constructivist orientation means that the interpretation of the data is closer to what is most commonly found in qualitative research. The assumption is made that there is not one truth or reality regarding practice-related issues but rather multiple realities and truths that often require innovative and unconventional methods to explore them. Practitioner research does not have the goal of producing knowledge that is valid outside of the specific setting in which the research study is conducted. The knowledge is a coproduction of the people involved in a particular social and historical context. However, because of the commonalities between settings regarding practice problems, interventions, professional conduct, and issues faced by clients/patients, a deeper understanding gained in one setting can inspire others in another setting to reflect on their work in new ways. This kind of generalizability by case comparison has been widely discussed in qualitative research and is part of the larger debate on what kinds of knowledge best promote human agency for social change (Starman, 2013; George, 2019)

1.2. The Benefits of Practitioner Research

Professional Development and Learning

In practice settings, research is usually conducted for pragmatic reasons, driven by the need to improve services. Practitioner research can be described as a strategic approach to advance professional development through experiential learning. The four phases of Kolb's (1984) experiential learning cycle are depicted in figure 1.1. In this cycle, reflective observation on a concrete experience can lead to abstract conceptualization followed by active experimentation and a new concrete experience. The cycle depicts the integration of subconscious emotional experiences with a cognitive conscious process, leading to the creation of new ideas and learned experiences. Practitioner research explicitly supports this process of empirically based learning.

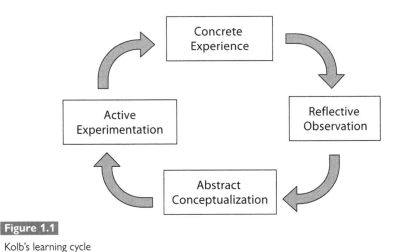

Figure 1.1

Kolb's learning cycle

Evidence-Based Decision-Making

Practitioners often face difficult situations that require making informed decisions—situations such as how to more effectively meet the needs of a specific client/patient through counseling, deciding what approach would work better under different scenarios, and how to address a conflict between a practitioner and a client/patient. Some of these situations can best be handled by making decisions based on past experience, observing standard protocols and practice norms, or seeking advice from a supervisor or other colleagues. However, as mentioned above, sometimes practitioners face systemic, recurrent issues where no clear course of action can be readily defined. Ways to address such issues can be developed systematically and empirically, thus providing an evidence base for future responses. In this way, practitioner research can be used as a powerful strategy to inform critical decision-making for improving services.

Evidence-based decision-making provides a useful framework for practitioner researchers in their attempt to integrate the best available research evidence with contextual and experiential evidence (figure 1.2). The framework allows for making adaptations to the research evidence during the implementation stage, especially when there are components that raise concern over the usefulness of the scientific evidence due to contextual and experiential practicalities. In other words, practitioner research can offer a solution to fit novel interventions in professional practice with high fidelity while making informed adaptations (Bania & Roebuck, 2018). In this way practitioner research can enhance the quality of decision-making in professional practice.

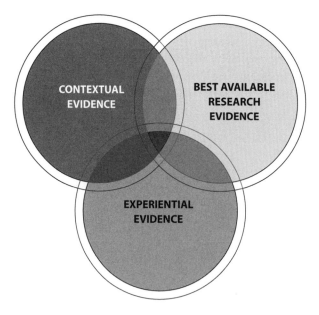

Figure 1.2

Evidence-based decision-making framework
(Centers for Disease Control and Prevention, n.d.)

Participation of All Stakeholders

Many practitioners are good at what they do, but the overall organization remains an abstraction for them. They work with a relatively small group of people with similar interests and responsibilities. It is with these teammates that they co-learn, find meaning in what they do, and create a sense of identity as a community. They learn practice norms within the context of their community through observation, dialogue, and reflection. Each member of a practice community has their own interpretation of what is happening in the practice environment; practitioner research can capture, map, and promote learning between the different perspectives (Cooper, 1993). More specifically, practitioner research can be used to create and enhance communities of practice in the following three dimensions, as described by Wenger (1998, p. 45): "a joint enterprise as understood and continually renegotiated by its members; the relationships of mutual engagement that binds members together into a social entity; and the shared repertoire of communal resources that members have developed over time."

Practitioner research is a form of participatory research (Wright, 2013) drawing from action research traditions. Stakeholders from health care and social services practice settings (e.g., service providers, clients and their families, management) need to be actively involved in designing and conducting research studies. According to Wright (2013), there are two main components to stakeholder participation: (1) the active involvement of the stakeholders for the purpose of improving their work or living situation; and (2) an equal partnership between all stakeholders for the mutual benefit of all. The participatory process ensures that the research project is relevant to the problem at hand so that the results can be translated into better services.

Practitioner research starts with identifying a practice problem that is perceived to be significant by both the practitioner and her organization and clientele. This is a very important precondition for developing a sense of ownership over the research process and the results. Previous studies show that a sense of research ownership is associated with the successful implementation of the results (Durlak & DuPre, 2008). This can lead to increased motivation for conducting robust and practical research as well as enhanced accountability among the health care and social work professionals.

Practitioner research studies can be conducted in partnership with affiliated or external academic institutions. However, the research must be co-owned by all parties involved and the practitioners must be active coresearchers, not merely in the role of recruiting participants or providing access to venues. Participation of people from different disciplines enriches the quality and potential impact of the studies. Multidisciplinary teamwork in research, however, is often challenging and requires a high level of coordination and accountability. The Practitioner Research Method presented in this book addresses the challenges to active involvement of people from different professions (e.g., allied health professions, nursing, social work, education) who are jointly working on and owning the process. Multidisciplinary practitioner research creates unique opportunities for comparing the results across different sites, validating or contributing to the body of literature, formulating new practice-based theories with broad applications, and identifying the need for further research.

Bridging the Gap between Evidence-Based Practice and Practice-Based Evidence

There is a gap and substantial delay between the discovery of new innovations and their implementation in practice settings. Through practitioner research, new research findings, theories, and evidence-based study results generated by academic institutions can be more rapidly and accurately implemented into daily practices while important aspects of the implementation process are also tested. In addition, practitioners can generate their own context-specific evidence for changes in their practice. In these ways, practice-based evidence is produced that can promote innovation in the respective field.

In practitioner research, practice and research are intertwined and cannot be separated from each other. It can be initially challenging for practitioners to maintain a balance between their roles as service providers and researchers. In practice settings, ethical and professional standards should always come first; research needs to be in line with these standards (Altrichter et al., 2008; Smeijsters et al., 2011). Practitioners' active involvement in research creates a reciprocity between research and practice in which research influences the routine professional practices and practice continuously changes the research agenda. For example, consider a nurse who is studying her patients' perceptions about the cleanliness of the hospital environment. A social desirability bias may lead to the underreporting of concerns on the part of the patients, and the underlying illnesses and duration of the hospitalizations may influence patients' expectations. Doing practitioner research on this topic requires a few back-and-forth pilot trials to learn the most practical approach to obtaining the most valid data for improving practice. What initially sounds like a relatively simple quality improvement initiative can have a larger impact leading to longer-term changes in professional practice in the hospital; the methods described in this book promote that kind of change. Practitioners need to be responsive to the needs and concerns of their clients/patients while carefully observing the practice environment in order to identify systematic patterns and interrelationships between underlying factors related to their research questions. Mastering the ability to observe carefully is challenging, as practitioners—like everyone else—are generally influenced by their own biases. But through practicing the research stance, practitioners become more aware of these biases and are more open to new information that may contradict their initial assumptions.

Example. A public health professional meets with a group of teenagers to learn about factors contributing to childhood obesity and weight gain. She believes that the availability of sweetened beverages in school cafeterias is the most important factor. As a result, she subconsciously spends most of the meeting time on that topic, which leaves her with less time to explore other factors.

Exercise 1. Practitioner Researchers' Dual Roles and Duty (see page 33)

Exercise 2. Research Ownership (see page 33)

The Practitioner Research Method

The Practitioner Research Method (Van der Donk & Van Lanen, 2019; Van der Donk & Van Lanen, 2020; Van der Donk et al., 2014) presented in this book comprises seven key components (figure 1.3) that can be applied to a variety of practitioner research designs. Although illustrated here with a sequence of arrows, the process of moving through the components is not always done in the same order; practitioners may choose to go back and forth between different stages if the original research questions and the way the practice problems are defined change, requiring going back and revising some of the activities. For example, most practitioners usually start by choosing a practice problem, collecting data, then analyzing the data according to a detailed research plan. However, the data analysis may suggest that changes are needed in both the formulation of practice problem and the research plan. Such changes may lead to the introduction of new variables that require collecting new data before moving on to the next step.

The components covering the Practitioner Research Cycle reflect a stepwise approach to planning and implementing a research project in a practice setting. Most practitioner research studies start with analyzing a practice problem followed by delving into the core issues and technical details. Together, the components guide the practitioner sequentially through the process of identifying and answering the research questions.

Furthermore, the additional Innovation Loop supports design research where the purpose of the research is to innovate. The Innovation Loop allows for designing the intervention and assessing and reassessing the emerging novel design by repeatedly collecting and analyzing new data. Innovative designs are usually informed by data collected through an array of simple and feasible methods, tools, and techniques (e.g. exit interviews, observation checklists, brainstorming). This process is similar to the concept of continuous quality improvement where a set of quality standards is defined for

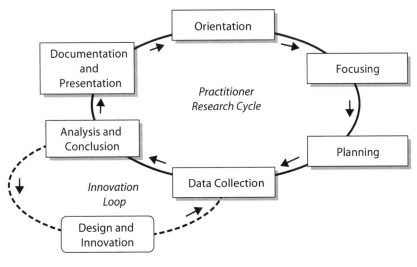

Figure 1.3

Components of the Practitioner Research Cycle and the Innovation Loop, which together make up our Practitioner Research Method

quality assurance and assessed on an ongoing basis (Kilo, 1998). In fact, practitioner research could be viewed as a specific approach to quality improvement in the interest of clients/patients, practitioners, and their organizations (Van der Donk et al., 2014).

All components of the Practitioner Research Method are described in the following sections in more detail.

Orientation

In the orientation stage, you will go through the process of exploring and mapping different practice problems and research questions. To do so, you will start by assessing your practice environment by, for example, reviewing available documentation and communicating with your colleagues and clients/patients. This assessment will deepen your understanding about any existing problems, including your understanding of those affected by the problems and the potential costs and benefits of addressing these problems. Exploring diverse perspectives and points of view will open your mind to new possibilities. Overall, the orientation component helps you acquire a well-founded overview of any problems in your professional practice and prepare you for the next stage of the method.

Focusing

This component is about zooming in on a significant practice problem in order to gain a better understanding about its possible causes and to identify critical questions that could only be answered through a practitioner research study. At this stage, you further review the scientific literature while continuing to assess your identified practice problem. This allows you to define and frame the practice problem by comparing and combining your experienced reality with scientific literature to substantiate your assumptions, a necessary step for learning more about what is known and about possible solutions. The beauty of focusing is that you are in control of shaping the direction of the research agenda and formulating the specific aims in the best way that suits the context of your professional practice.

Planning

At this stage, you have the fundamental information you need to select the most robust yet practical methodological approach for designing your practitioner research study. First, you will be introduced to a variety of techniques and ideas for choosing the best research activities—from a menu of options—that could provide valid data to answer different types of research questions. Second, you will plan your research activities, such as participant recruitment, timing and duration of the study, and quality assurance and control measures. Lastly, your planning will include budgeting: calculating the amount of funding you would need and documenting any in-kind resources or support that you could generate. In the first two stages of the Practitioner Research Method, you prepare for the research project by selecting the research topic, collecting the necessary information, and creating the building blocks to plan the study. In the planning stage, you learn how to use your best judgement to put all you have acquired to good use.

Data Collection

A logical step after planning the study is to conduct the research and collect the data. At this stage, you will learn about common tools and methods that are used for data collection in practice settings, such as mind mapping, systematic observation, role-playing, storytelling, and so on. You will learn how to use standard tools, such as questionnaires, checklists, charts, and interview guides. In addition, you will learn how to decide whether to use available tools, or if you need to modify existing tools or even create your own instruments, based on your needs.

Analysis and Conclusion

At this stage, you consider data management techniques that could help you prepare for conducting data analysis. There are practical data analysis methods you can choose from according to the nature of your research questions and specific aims, as well as effective strategies for discussing and sharing the results to inform thoughtful discussions and drawing conclusions.

Design and Innovation

This component is only relevant to practitioner research studies in which the development of an intervention is the goal. An intervention could be a new treatment method, an educational brochure, a practice protocol, or something of that nature. This type of study is called design research and is conducted in two phases. In phase one, descriptive research methods are used to identify important principles to design an intervention to solve your practice problem. In phase two, you design the intervention and test its effectiveness by conducting a small experiment or pilot. You use this data to improve the intervention and then test it again, collecting and analyzing data for the purpose of making further improvements. You repeat this Innovation Loop until you are satisfied with the intervention's performance.

Documentation and Presentation

The final component of the Practitioner Research Method is where you document your study and disseminate the results. Documenting your best experiences and lessons learned can save scarce resources by preventing systematic mistakes and enhancing the effectiveness of services. Further, you can claim credit for improving your professional practice through effective documentation and presentation. Some practitioner research studies are only relevant to the local practice setting and a close circle of associates and clients. Other studies have broader appeal and could benefit many more practice settings than your own. To facilitate broader dissemination and implementation, you will need to be engaged in activities that help you identify opportunities for professional networking, presentations, and publications. Documentation and presentation are integral parts of every practitioner research study and need to be planned according to the specific parameters and resources.

An Example from the Field

The following simplified example of the entire Practitioner Research Method is provided to clarify the iterative nature of practitioner research and the range of research activities relevant to a selected practice problem.

Orientation

Parents of students in an after-school program participated in a satisfaction survey. They reported high levels of satisfaction with staff members' professional skills and competency, but several parents expressed concerns over the safety of their children. The program director called for a brainstorming meeting with her staff in order to gain more insights into the problem and generate a mind map on how the problem is collectively viewed (see chapter 2 for more details on mind maps). Then she invited the parents to a meeting with the aim of having an in-depth discussion about their safety concerns and to find out how they want the problem to be addressed.

Focusing

In preparation for the meeting, the director read journal articles from credible sources on child safety in after-school programs. At the meeting, the parents' chief concern was about the perceived low level of supervision during outdoor playtimes. This was somewhat disappointing to the director, as the program intended to foster independence in children by giving them more freedom of movement while observing them from a reasonable distance. The program director noticed that the parents had not been fully informed about the policy. However, she took this very seriously and drafted the following research question: "How can we enhance and maintain parents' satisfaction with child safety measures taken by the program during outdoor playtime while maintaining the growth of the children's independence?"

Planning

The program director generated an initial list of potential research activities that could help answer the question. Then, she scheduled a few meetings with her staff and made a plan to observe the playground multiple times during the outdoor playtimes. In preparation for such activities, she set aside specific dates and times for developing the agenda of the staff meetings, an observation checklist, and a documentation plan.

Data Collection

During the meetings, many staff members agreed with the parents' safety concerns. They mentioned a few specific playground areas that are not fully childproof and that contain dangerous blind spots that are difficult for the staff to monitor. This is partly because the playground was designed to have places for children to hide for hide-and-seek and other games. During the observation times, the program director paid attention to how much children were enjoying their time while documenting the number of supervising staff and marking their locations. She surveyed the area and made notes about potentially unsafe places and behaviors that could result in children injuring themselves or each other. Lastly, she noticed that the staff might not be able to oversee the whole area, but also that the children are often very quick in reporting conflicts and accidents. These observations gave the program director some novel ideas for better staffing, better use of technology and surveillance cameras, and engaging children in more responsible behaviors.

Analysis and Conclusion

After conducting the research activities, the program director felt that she had been able to acquire enough data for a detailed description of the practice problem. Now it was time to analyze the data, reflect on the results, and then suggest potential responses and their required resources. She engaged her staff and a few parents in the discussion to make sure that the planned changes were aligned with everyone's expectations.

The program director invited a playground designer, three staff members, and two parents to a meeting to discuss the strategic goals and basic principles of improving the safety of the playground. The three main characteristics of a good intervention were identified as follows:

1. A minimum of two staff members is needed to oversee a playgroup.
2. The challenging play areas need to be maintained and increased while the safety of the playground is enhanced.
3. The cost of making changes should be affordable for the program.

Innovation Loop

After a few rounds of brainstorming and reflection, the team generated some promising ideas, such as staff members walking along a marked route during playtime rather than standing at fixed stations and the program convening information sessions to inform and engage parents in a discussion about the program's playtime policy of instilling a strong sense of independence and responsibility in their children. These ideas were implemented over a period of a few months with careful attention to the details, and the program director and her colleagues had to revise the original plan based on the pilot data. Two months following implementation, another satisfaction survey was administered that showed a significant increase in parents' satisfaction.

Documentation and Presentation

The program director presented the findings to the parents and the board of education. In addition, she wrote a short report about the study that was published in a practice magazine and in the program's monthly newsletter. One of the staff members created a short video about the whole initiative, which was posted on the program's website and social media. The positive publicity resulting from the initiative increased the rating of the program, which led to more recognition and economic benefits for the staff and the program.

This example demonstrates the dynamic nature of practitioner research in an educational or pedagogical setting. The selection of this setting was intentional to make it possible for everyone to understand the key components and the overall concept. The same principles can then be followed in health care and social services settings.

Exercise 3. The Stages of the Practitioner Research Method (see page 34)

Similar to other forms of systematic inquiry, certain principles need to be followed and maintained in order to ensure the integrity of practitioner research. The quality of practitioner research depends on the validity and reliability of its findings, and there are a number of useful guidelines we can give for improving these basic quality control measures of your research.

Validity

The noun "valid" is often used interchangeably with "genuine" and "sound." In quantitative research (a positivist research approach, remember), validity applies to whether the tools are able to genuinely measure what they intend to measure and if the results are sound and generalizable in other similar situations. The validity of the tools and the data in a research study is often called *internal validity*, while the generalizability of the findings to other settings is referred to as *external validity*. In other words, internal validity is about the quality of the research findings, and external validity refers to the usefulness of the findings outside of their original research context. Overall, internal and external validity as defined here depend on the robustness of the design, the validity of instruments, the quality of the implementation, and the inclusion of diverse perspectives and settings. A strong research design establishes a controlled environment where different hypotheses are tested and the effects of possible confounders are minimized.

As described earlier, practitioner research follows a constructivist paradigm. The definitions of validity and reliability as found in quantitative research are often explained differently. In real-life practice settings, services are often delivered under less-than-optimal circumstances, which can dilute and compromise the ultimate intended outcomes. And in practitioner research it is more about how to improve the effectiveness of services under real-life conditions rather than measuring the efficacy of services under ideal circumstances. Therefore, a different set of validity criteria are needed.

Anderson et al. (2007) and Herr and Anderson (2015) describe practitioner research outcome and process validity according to its unique characteristics, such as the insider status of the researchers, the centrality of action, the iterative nature of reflection on actions, and the close relationship between research and practice. *Outcome validity* is defined as the extent to which the problem that inspired research is addressed as the result of conducting the study. In other words, the outcome validity is as simple as whether the research was successful in generating the intended outcome of improving the practice. However, the word "success" often needs explanation, as in practitioner research the questions usually transform into a new set of questions, and the original practice problem gets redefined following the initial inquiries and participation of other colleagues. *Process validity* is a concept that assesses the extent of framing and resolving practice problems in a participatory and iterative manner allowing for several rounds of ongoing reflection and co-learning among all parties involved. Inclusion of multiple perspectives is a strategy for protecting against the generation of simplistic and self-serving evidence with major flaws and errors. In reality, a high level of process validity should lead to better outcome validity.

One important domain of process validity is *democratic validity*, referring to the level of involvement and collaboration among internal stakeholders. *Catalytic validity* is another domain of process validity that refers to the extent of orientation, focus, and energy created by the research and expressed as a sense of enthusiasm among the team members for knowing more and moving forward. Lastly, *dialogical validity* is the extent of internal or external stakeholders' and partners' involvement in providing peer review and reflection on the process. The aforementioned criteria can provide a template for defining relevant metrics and tools—mostly qualitative—to increase the internal validity of practitioner research studies.

Understanding Outcome and Process Validity

The following example is provided to help better illustrate issues related to outcome and process validity in practitioner research. Relevant concepts that have been discussed so far in this chapter are in bold.

> The curriculum committee of a school of nursing intends to increase student enrollment in the practitioner research course (**original intended outcome**). The idea was presented by the primary instructor based on the potential benefits of practitioner research in enriching students' research training and actively engaging them in real-life professional practices. But few students have been taking the course since it was first offered two years ago (**practice problem**). After extensive discussions, the primary instructor accepted the task of conducting a practitioner research study on this subject. She put together a diverse team to further explore the issues and drafted the following **initial research question** for the project: How can we increase students' enrollment in the practitioner research course?
>
> Next, the primary instructor invited the following individuals to a meeting: two former and two current students, two colleagues, two representatives from partner local clinics, and two patients from previous projects conducted by the former students (**initial process**). At the meeting, she conducted a brainstorming exercise around the following questions: What has been your level of experience with and involvement in practitioner research? What are the most useful aspects of your experience? How would you improve the quality of your past exposure? Everyone had the chance to participate and all comments were documented on flipcharts without participants criticizing and arguing among each other. At the end, the participants were happy about their contributions, but some important opposing opinions and ideas emerged.
>
> The primary instructor presented a plan for summarizing and organizing everyone's points as well as having a few other meetings on specific topics to resolve any potential conflicts. She added that after a few rounds of discussion, a shared decision would be made about making possible changes to the research question, the practice problem, and the intended outcome (**process validity**). Some participants mentioned that they want to have a more prominent role in shaping the agenda and summarizing the results of the meeting. The primary instructor liked the idea and agreed to involve them in the process. In addition, she promised to share draft documents so everyone could have a chance to propose changes and

modify the plan (**democratic validity**). The team was satisfied with the agreement and the plan was carried out accordingly.

After a few meetings, the team developed a consensus around the important aspects of the project. First, they agreed that the students' enrollment in the practitioner research course should be viewed more broadly in the context of their awareness of the course, the content of the course, the quality of training, the relationship with partner hospitals and clinics, the adequacy of logistical support, and the readiness of the practice sites to be involved in research. Therefore, the aim expanded from focusing on increasing students' enrollment in the course to improving buy-in for conducting practitioner research from the students, faculty, and partner organizations (**revised outcome**). Therefore, the practice problem was redefined as the "limited awareness of and less than optimal quality of practitioner research in the school and collaborating sites" (**redefined practice problem**). Subsequently, a **new set of research questions** were identified: How to more effectively market the course to the students? How to enhance the quality of the training? How to increase the number of partner organizations and strengthen the school's relationship with them? What logistical support is required? How to increase the buy-in from participating sites for conducting practitioner research projects?

The new agenda was perceived to be both enabling and more relevant to the needs of the collaborating team, evidenced by the increased number of volunteers, a strong sense of enthusiasm, more positive feedback, more willingness to participate, and the increased level of in-kind contributions (**catalytic validity**). Furthermore, new task forces were formed around answering the research questions more relevant to each group (i.e., faculty, students, practitioners). Each group formed their own leadership structure and shared their findings with other groups and actively solicited their feedback (**dialogical validity**). As a result of the improved process, the following changes occurred:

- Students took an active role in producing useful promotional materials about the course and distributing them among their peers. The quality of the materials and the marketing campaign were enhanced with feedback from former and current students as well as the school's staff. In addition, the office of student affairs used the materials to further promote the course.

- The curriculum committee reviewed the contents of the course and approved revisions suggested by the instructor based on feedback from her former students, partner organizations, and former clients.

- The practice sites made important recommendations for having mutually beneficial relationships with the school. After a few revisions, the terms of the collaboration were accepted and written into a formal memorandum of agreement between each site and the school of nursing.

- One year after the start of the project, the practitioner research course was rated as one of the most useful courses and became a mandatory course for all undergraduate nursing students. The number of participating practice sites increased over time, and several health care practitioners from participating sites started conducting their own practitioner research projects (**outcome validity**).

The external validity of practitioner research (i.e., the generalizability of the results to other settings) is not as important as internal validity. This is mainly because the knowledge and insights acquired through practitioner research are highly specific to the context. In most cases, it is not expected that the results of practitioner research studies will be generalizable to other settings. However, practitioner research can often provide important practice-based evidence on how to implement scientific interventions resulting from studies with high internal validity, often referred to as *efficacy trials* (Glasgow et al., 2003). Such studies are conducted under controlled experimental conditions and have been proven useful in generating positive outcomes, but the applicability of such studies under real-life settings are limited due to their low external validity. Through practitioner research, such evidence-based practices can be implemented with attention to overall feasibility, the core aspects of the interventions, and innovative ways for optimizing their effects under the specific context of professional practice. The results of such studies can enrich the overall understanding of the intervention in different contexts and can be used by other practitioners in their effort to adopt such evidence in their own organizations.

Reliability

In our daily life, we usually use "reliability" to mean "honesty" and "integrity." In quantitative research, reliability is defined as the consistency level of the results when the study is repeated using the same methodology by different researchers. In other words, highly reliable scientific research studies are the ones that are replicable and repeatable over time, and that can generate consistent results. One example could be the reliability of a questionnaire, which can be assessed by the same group of participants taking and retaking the survey. Responses generated by a reliable research questionnaire would be similar when used repeatedly over time. This attribute is often referred to as the *stability of the instrument*. It is obvious that without reliable methods and tools, research studies cannot be valid and generalizable. That's why reliability criteria—similar to validity criteria—are quality measures of the worthiness of scientific evidence generated by research.

Golafshani (2003) makes an argument about the importance of redefining the concept of reliability for qualitative research while adhering to its most important function of testing the integrity and robustness of the research. In contrast to quantitative studies, whose main purpose is to describe events and test hypotheses, the primary goal of qualitative studies is to generate understanding by exploring different phenomena and constructing plural realities. Therefore, reliability in qualitative research often refers to the *credibility* of the study and *dependability* of the results rather than the results' replicability and generalizability. Similar approaches are needed to understand and define reliability criteria for practitioner research. According to the definition, the primary purpose of practitioner research is to generate practical knowledge using a wide range of feasible qualitative and quantitative methods conducted by the practice community to improve the quality of the services at individual and institutional levels. To attain this goal, reliable tools and methods need to be utilized as much as possible in the real-life context of practice settings. But at the end, a reliable practitioner research study is the type of systematic inquiry that results in practice-based evidence and products that are credible, dependable, and useful.

Guidelines in Achieving Validity and Reliability

Guideline 1: Be Attentive to Bias

To enhance validity and reliability, we first need to understand and identify factors that negatively affect them. Confounder variables can negatively affect the validity and accuracy of the findings. In addition, unexpected events could lead to undesirable interactions among the study variables. For example, imagine a situation where you are conducting a job-satisfaction survey; meanwhile, a few hours before, management announced major budget cuts that will financially affect many of the employees. Such an event can significantly impact employees' expressions of job satisfaction and the reliability of your results. Lastly, several other methodological errors and research biases could compromise the reliability and validity of your study:

- *Selection bias* is when some of your clients and patients are not participating in the study due to factors such as the timing of your research, logistical challenges like lack of transportation and childcare, and lack of incentives.

- *Social desirability bias* is when an honest answer to a question is perceived as not being desirable because of the possibility of negative reactions and consequences. For example, when a practitioner asks a question about a patient's satisfaction with a service that has just been provided, the patient might see it as more socially desirable to praise the practitioner rather than state any concerns.

- *Information bias* is the result of measurement errors that could be as simple as mistaken observations and misclassifications or the participants not understanding the questions asked.

- *Intervention bias* is when, as part of the research process, your patients receive additional services and interventions that could cloud their perceptions of the services that you are trying to study or improve.

Guideline 2: Triangulate Sources, Methods, and Researchers

Triangulation refers to collecting data using more than one approach in order to enhance the validity and reliability of the study (Bryman, 2004). The concept of triangulation was first introduced by Webb et al. (1966), who mentioned that uncertainties around the research findings could be greatly reduced if the results are confirmed by two or more independent measurements. The concept can be defined as using data from various sources (multiple perspectives), collecting data through different methods, and including other researchers in data collection and analysis (figure 1.4).

Triangulation of sources is when you collect data from various sources to compare results from different respondents in order to cross-validate the accuracy of findings. For example, if most youth enrolled in a summer program reported being highly pleased with the program, you would expect the results of similar surveys or focus group discussions conducted with parents, teachers, and staff to confirm this finding. If not, this may raise a question about the trustworthiness of the results from the youth and require further exploration of the situation to better understand it. Triangulation

Triangulation

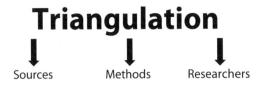

Sources   Methods   Researchers

Figure 1.4

Triangulation applies to collecting data across numerous sources, methods, and researchers in order to enhance validity and reliability of a study

of sources could also involve examining various secondary data such as historical documents, meeting notes, annual reports, service statistics, and published articles. In addition to expanding the knowledge base, the purpose here is to determine if findings from different sources are or are not in agreement.

Triangulation of methods refers to utilizing different methodological approaches for collecting data and interpreting the results due to the unique methodological strengths and weaknesses that using each method would bring to the table. For example, observing your colleagues in a natural situation could give you a different type of data compared to asking them questions in a private interview. Furthermore, quantitative surveys are designed to answer questions regarding the magnitude and scope of an event, while a qualitative focus group discussion would explore the rationale and underlying processes leading to the event. Therefore, by using multiple methods for collecting data, you will be able to both benefit from the complementary nature of your findings and validate the accuracy and trustworthiness of your overall results.

Researcher triangulation is a concept that applies to a situation where multiple researchers work separately on the same study. This approach could be a powerful way to identify areas where researchers may have varying results. The results could be different simply because of human error, such as entering data incorrectly. Since it is less likely for different people to make the same mistake in a large database, comparing the researchers' outputs could quickly discover such mistakes. However, there are other types of discrepancies that could happen because of lack of clarity, misunderstanding, and following different criteria. Involving multiple researchers in certain tasks, such as coding qualitative data, interpreting the results, and so on, can help identify such areas of discrepancy. Lastly, people with different backgrounds would bring different perspectives and view phenomena from unique angles. Involving a diverse group of researchers in interpreting the results can maximize the effects and usefulness of the findings for professional practice.

Exercise 4. Triangulation (see page 34)

Guideline 3: Actively Involve a Diverse Group of Stakeholders

Building on the idea of triangulation, active involvement of a diverse group of stakeholders, too, is necessary to ensure the relevance, quality, and effectiveness of practitioner research. Stakeholders such as patients, colleagues, administrators, and policy makers view practitioner research from different perspectives. For example, a practitioner's primary motivation for conducting a study could be to make services more convenient, while a patient's primary interest could be the cost-effectiveness of the services. On the other hand, administrators usually view research from an organizational perspective, and policy makers are more interested in how the results will inform new policies.

Involving key stakeholders early in the process increases the validity of the study by enhancing the knowledge pool and the odds of results being put into practice from shared ownership of the research. To make this process work, you would need to effectively communicate the significance of your study, the rationale for making changes, as well as the potential consequences. Here transparent communication is key to minimize ambiguity and misunderstandings and to build a solid foundation for a trusting relationship. Overall validity and rigor of practitioner research highly depends on the extent of your collaborations and the quality of your relationship with different stakeholders. Effective inclusion of stakeholders requires organization, honesty, humility, knowledge sharing, and equal access to information. It will be crucial to keep an open mind and seriously consider every perspective that your team members bring to the table.

Guideline 4: Explore the Practice Problem, the Organization, and the Scientific and Professional Literature

The practice problem that you intend to study is the product of a dynamic ecological system that clients, practitioners, colleagues, the organization, and the larger sociopolitical system all play roles in creating and maintaining. The more you understand your practice problem, the more you will be able to design a relevant research study to address the problem. You can start exploring the practice problem by conducting a problem analysis that includes, but is not limited to, talking with different stakeholders, reviewing relevant resources and data, presenting your ideas, soliciting feedback, reviewing historical information about the organization, and reviewing relevant professional and scientific literature.

The problem analysis is an important step that allows you to view the problem in a broader context and explore its underlying themes and related factors. Without a good orientation to the practice problem, it would be very hard to conduct successful practitioner research. Furthermore, practitioner research studies should be aligned with existing procedures, protocols, and organizational policies. Therefore, it is important to explore the specific features of the organization, such as geographic location; partnerships with other organizations, clients, and patients; funding mechanisms; leadership structure; and organizational culture. You can do this yourself by conducting interviews with key individuals in different positions to capture and incorporate various organizational perspectives related to your practice problem. For instance, think about the layout of a waiting area: a patient might be concerned about her privacy in the area; the receptionist may want to have an unobstructed view; an administrator views the area with attention to compliance with legal requirements; a child looks for play materials; and a janitor may wish that the area is easy to clean. Information you gain here could be used later to enhance support for your research.

Lastly, a good practitioner researcher always stays current with the literature by reading scientific and professional articles relevant to his practice problem. Every article is written through a specific disciplinary perspective, which can illuminate important aspects unknown to the practitioner. In addition, through a comprehensive literature review, one can learn a lot from the technical and scientific aspects of the problem that can prevent redundancies and making similar mistakes. Overall, the validity and reliability/credibility of your study have a direct relationship with your level of knowledge of and experience with the problem, the organization, and the scientific literature.

1.5. Types of Practitioner Research Questions

The design of your practitioner research study ultimately depends on the type of research question that you ask. Here we will describe five different types of practitioner research questions, namely descriptive, defining, comparative, evaluative, and explanatory.

Descriptive questions: These questions seek to either describe the current state of affairs regarding the issue under study or provide information about needed improvements. Needs assessments are a common form of research that falls into this category. Some examples are:

- What kind of support do the people in our health center who are living with cancer need?
- Where do homeless people find help in our city?
- Is there a problem with violence in our school?
- What information do refugees in our region need about health and social services?
- What are the most important places for members of our community to meet and socialize?
- What do our young people know about drugs and their effects?
- What are the major strengths of our organization?
- What kind of youth-friendly training materials are needed for tobacco education?
- What are some of the unmet needs and training gaps in the sex education curriculum?

Defining questions: These questions seek to define an important idea or concept from the perspective of a particular group of people or several different groups of people. The definitions of important terms such as "poverty," "homelessness," or "refugee" most often come from people who aren't directly affected by these issues, and the definitions can be associated with negative connotations. A focus of participatory research projects can be defining an issue from the perspective of those affected. Some examples are:

- What does it mean to be healthy from the perspective of people with rheumatoid arthritis?
- The people in our district are described as being poor. How do we define ourselves? Do we see ourselves as being poor? What do we mean by the word "poor"?
- A goal of our clinic is to be patient-centered. How do our patients define that concept?

- What is a "safe neighborhood" from the perspective of those who live in this district?
- How do youth in our neighborhood define violence?

Comparative questions: These questions compare one thing to another in order to find out what the differences and similarities are. Some examples are:

- How healthy are homeless people compared to others in our community?
- What programs do girls need help with compared to boys?
- What kind of information do new parents get about raising their children from pediatricians compared to the information they get from parents in their neighborhood?
- In which district of our city are people healthiest?
- Which form of counseling most helps youth with their drug problems, peer counseling or outreach work by social workers?

Evaluative questions: These questions aim at determining the value of a particular action or service, usually in terms of the goals that were set by those conducting the action or service. Evaluation questions are often focused on the effectiveness of a particular action. Some examples are:

- How successful were our efforts to mobilize residents in taking action for better housing conditions?
- Does our counseling program help women who have experienced domestic violence?
- To what extend has our neighborhood action resulted in safer streets?
- How successful have we been able to reach more older people living alone?
- To what extend has the health of our community improved over the last year since we have launched our health campaign?

Explanatory questions: These questions are usually focused on finding out why something is the way it is. Finding out why certain policies or practices are in place can be key in knowing how best to take action for improving a situation. Some examples are:

- Why are people in our neighborhood less healthy than people in other neighborhoods?
- Why have all our efforts to stop youth from dropping out of school failed?
- Why is the new family center so successful?
- Why do so few people come to our drop-in center?
- How can we explain the rise in violence in this district over the last year?
- What is the reason for the large number of people developing respiratory problems in our building?

The various types of questions may be combined. For example, in an evaluation of a certain service (evaluative question) we may be interested in finding out if there is a difference between men and women in terms of effectiveness (comparative question). We may also want to find out why the service was effective in some cases and not in others (explanatory question). Or in describing the types of assistance homeless people need (descriptive question) we may be interested in how the homeless people define what they consider to be a useful service (defining question).

Exercise 5. Types of Research Questions (see page 34)

1.6. The Scope of Practitioner Research Projects

Practitioner research can be conducted at multiple levels, depending on the goals and focus of the study. These levels can be divided into five categories: individual, departmental, organizational, interorganizational, and community.

Level	Possible overarching goal	Possible focus of the study
Individual	Improving the quality and effectiveness of services, enhancing clients' satisfaction	Roles and responsibilities of the practitioner and his/her expected impact
Departmental	Improving the quality of services, policy and procedures, and overall effectiveness and productivity	Departmental polices, administrative structure, processes, functions, and hallmarks of success
Organizational	Improving the capacity, the cost-effectiveness, the level of funding and revenues, coordination between different departments, and satisfaction among clients and staff	Organizational polices, cultural norms, administrative structure, internal processes, functions, and hallmarks of success
Interorganizational	Improving care networks and systems, collaboration among different organizations/agencies, policy and regulations, sustainability and effectiveness of professional practice	Professional practice networks and their leadership structure; needs, functions, and strategic objectives; formal partnerships and interdisciplinary research
Community	Identifying community needs and assets; building and maintaining trusting relationships with service providers; designing and implementing sustainable community-based programs and initiatives; improving health and wellness	Community programs, policy, structure and dynamics, funding and resources, leadership, health and wellness, culture, and economics

1.7. Practitioner Research in Health Care and Social Service Settings

Conducting research in professional practice settings is not easy or free of challenges. Health care and social service settings have special characteristics that could pose limitations on and present obstacles for conducting practitioner research. And there are lessons to be learned that may provide insights on how practitioner research could be used as a strategic approach—rather than simply as an additional professional activity—for addressing practice problems. Practitioner research, as discussed earlier, can be conducted at different levels (e.g. client services, organizational structure, policy) with important benefits at each level. All things considered, there are innovative strategies for generating support and incentives for conducting practitioner research. The goal is to create a long-term vision for enhancing the capacity of the organization for conducting research by first focusing on pragmatic needs, such as quality improvements, that pave the road for addressing strategic needs, which are often reflected in organizational policies and culture. And finally, the ethical aspects of conducting research in practice settings along with examples from the field will help clarify these issues.

Special Characteristics of Community, Health Care, and Social Service Settings

Practitioner research in community and professional practice settings such as health care and social services has the potential for widespread improvement in the health and social well-being of the population. "Community" is defined as a group that unifies its members around a shared identity (Israel et al., 1998). We often consider communities to be defined by the geographic locations in which their members live, work, play, or pray together. With the invention of modern communication technologies, however, communities can also form virtually around shared identities such as sexual orientation, health conditions, ethnicity, and so on. Practitioners often need to go outside their practice organizations to meet their clients in their own communities for marketing and outreach purposes. In addition, community can be an ideal place for offering many health care and social work services.

Numerous assets exist in the context of a community, such as local businesses, government organizations, schools, nonprofit organizations, faith-based organizations, and highly motivated and knowledgeable individuals. Such assets have the potential to enhance the quality and effectiveness of services if better utilized by practitioners working in health care and social services organizations. Conducting practitioner research in community settings requires building trusting relationships with key players and negotiating a shared mission. Unlike organizational settings, member interactions in the context of their own communities are often based on moral codes and accepted cultural and social norms rather than through formal procedures and contracts. A certain level of dialogue always exists in an ongoing manner among community members, and motivations to act are based on the collective wisdom of what is needed.

Community members have different levels of access to and control over existing resources and they form social networks to share and utilize the resources. The informal and not-so-obvious structures of community settings can pose critical challenges and compromise the feasibility of conducting practitioner research or enable and enhance practitioner research. Through effective engagement with community stakeholders, the quality and sustainability of interventions can be substantially improved while the cost of the interventions is significantly reduced. We will discuss further details about how to conduct practitioner research in community settings in the next section.

Like communities, health care settings can also be defined according to a common set of basic characteristics, such as fundamental culture and professional norms; common bureaucratic systems, rules, and regulations; and similar challenges although with different scopes and intensity. Health care settings can also differ significantly according to their size (ranging from small physician practices to large specialized hospitals), level of services (i.e., providing primary, secondary, or tertiary preventive services), patient characteristics (e.g., sociodemographic, health condition), type of services (e.g., pediatrics, family medicine, geriatrics), and type of programs (e.g., public, private for profit, private nonprofit). After graduation, physicians and other practitioners are usually expected to make diagnostic, treatment, and recovery decisions on a case-by-case basis, relying more on their own experiences—and their peers'—rather than new evidence-based practices documented in systematic reviews (Gabbay & le May, 2016).

Since practitioners usually prefer guidelines offering a voluntary set of parameters over those with more rigid and prescribed mandates, it has been historically difficult to implement new scientific evidence into professional practice. And as much as practitioners often expect that their professional autonomy will be respected, practice organizations are usually set up according to bureaucratic hierarchies in which those in higher positions traditionally have more decision-making power and control over procedures. This can lead to conflicts between highly educated frontline practitioners and high-level administrators of their organization.

Conflicts can become further complicated by levels of uncertainty inherent to clinical practice, such as variability in treatment outcomes, resources, and psychological aspects of interactions between practitioners and their clients (Brownson, 2012, p. 405–7). In other words, sometimes the options and the path forward are not clear. Lastly, practitioners often face challenges such as working in environments with less than optimal resources, support, and clarity. Practitioner research can address many of the challenges mentioned here by empowering providers to investigate their own work and integrate the scientific and validated practice-based data needed for making informed decisions.

That brings us to social services settings, which are usually the base for providing services within complex networks of care to underserved clients disproportionately affected by various disparities. Social services programs can be characterized using five domains introduced by Damschroder et al. (2009) as a framework for implementing evidence-based practices into complex settings: the services provided, involved practitioners, the organizational context, the external environment, and the implementation process.

"Social services" is a broad term often used to cover a wide range of social, health, and well-being services offered both by health care systems as well as nonmedical sectors, such as criminal justice, housing, and welfare departments. Some examples of social services include, but are not limited to, child maltreatment investigation and responses, juvenile justice services (e.g., delinquency prevention, counseling, and residential services), welfare services to needy families, nutrition assistance programs, public housing assistance, long-term care, and services for victims of domestic violence.

Practitioners involved in providing social services assume a variety of roles, such as case manager, community organizer, counselor, social service investigator, and facilitator of support groups, among others. Some individuals and families interact frequently with their social service providers over a long period of time. For many such families, their social services case manager is their gatekeeper connecting them to other services and fulfilling the role of a primary care provider. To be successful, practitioners need to interact and collaborate with many external players, such as those from organizations that provide wraparound services. The problems that practitioners are expected to address are often multifaceted, requiring interventions at more than one level and often under the jurisdiction of multiple departments. Social services practitioners and their respective organizations need to work closely as a team along with their clients to find innovative solutions to improve their clients' situations.

Practitioner Research as a Strategic Approach for Improving Health Care and Social Services

Practitioner research should be viewed as a strategic approach—rather than an add-on assignment—for improving professional practice. Many of the challenges that health care and social services practitioners face in their professional practices can be effectively addressed by conducting successful practitioner research over a reasonable time period. Here we describe how practitioner research can improve your professional practice by removing hard-to-address obstacles, saving you time, saving organizational resources, and improving the overall impact of services. In the next section, we will give you some ideas on how to start doing practitioner research more effectively (and maintain your engagement with it) so you can reap the rewards and enjoy the results.

As discussed earlier, professional practice is filled with situations where making decisions relies on the knowledge, experience, and judgment of the practitioners about what's needed for each specific client. The main reason for practitioners not favoring highly detailed protocols with prescribed mandates is that many such mandates may not exactly work the way they are prescribed. For example, a practitioner may find a protocol inappropriate in which an age limit has been set as a qualifying criterion for receiving a medical procedure if many of her older patients could significantly benefit from it. In this scenario, practitioner research could be a powerful tool to justify clinical decisions made on the ground with documented results of their benefits for the clients. In fact, the conflict between respecting practitioners' expertise and autonomy and the top-down approach to implementing evidence-based practices can be resolved through practitioner research.

By taking the driver's seat in research, practitioners can maintain their sense of autonomy over the study design, implementation, and interpretation of the results in a way that is most appropriate and relevant to their professional practice. Practitioner research studies often combine providers' experiential knowledge with empirical data, which can result in even stronger evidence that is difficult to ignore. Such evidence can reduce the level of professional uncertainty about care decisions and lead to an enhanced sense of confidence among the service providers. The empowering impact of data can further strengthen frontline practitioners' positions in negotiating with higher-level administrators and regulatory agencies about protocols and treatments that make the most sense.

This is an important precondition for creating a more participatory learning environment with the shared vision of doing what's best for the professional practice and communities you intend to serve. Through practitioner research, health care and social services practitioners can enhance their position to a level where they can effectively examine their roles and responsibilities while forming powerful partnerships with internal and external stakeholders. This can lead to enhanced capacity and readiness for having a more meaningful impact both at the individual and organizational levels. In a way, practitioner research—if well understood and applied—can help you mobilize everyone around you toward shaping a glorious future . . . rather than remaining in the status quo or in a state of limbo.

Generating Support and Room to Maneuver

Despite the promise of practitioner research, you still need to convince others in your specific setting that your planned research project will result in a reasonable return on investment. This requires knowledge and expertise in how to conduct a successful research project, an interesting topic for the research, support from your colleagues and management, trusting relationships with key stakeholders, and logistical support and resources. The Practitioner Research Method will help you critically appraise your work environment, identify potential practice problems, and generate promising ideas to address them. Your success in generating support depends on both the merits of your ideas and how you present them.

Of central importance is the kind of needs that you intend to address in your research. We distinguish between two types of needs: *pragmatic needs* versus *strategic needs* (Moser, 1989). Pragmatic needs refer to demands for improving quality that are not controversial and that do not require changing the culture, norms, or values in the organization. Strategic needs, on the other hand, raise critical issues requiring fundamental organizational change, for example, involving issues of access, equity, or fairness. To illustrate, improving the effectiveness of a counseling program in an agency providing family services would generally be considered a pragmatic issue. However, identifying access barriers to African American families in obtaining counseling at the agency raises strategic issues that may involve examining racial biases on the part of staff. In practitioner research you can always identify nonsensitive practice problems and those that are more political, controversial, or sensitive. Some practitioners might be tempted to first tackle the latter. However, a research project addressing such issues may be doomed to fail due to a lack of support from colleagues, the management level, or funders. Therefore, it is wise to first focus on your organization's pragmatic needs when embarking on practitioner research. The positive results can provide a basis for approaching topics in the future requiring deeper organizational change. This approach uses the power of practitioner research to gradually increase your room to maneuver and to build your organization's readiness for change.

Exercise 6. Research Context of Your Organization (see page 35)

Ethical Considerations

Practitioner research can be conducted at multiple levels, as already described. Regardless of the scope, however, there are several ethical considerations that need to be considered. In general, ethical conduct of research involving human subjects requires meeting three basic ethical considerations: (1) you need to make sure that the participants are adequately informed while respecting their privacy; (2) you need to carefully listen to participants' concerns about the confidentiality of their data and make sure that their decision to participate is voluntary and without any coercion or undue influence; and (3) you need to make sure the participants fully understand the potential risks and benefits of (as well as alternatives to) participating in your study.

In professional practice settings, the expectation of clients/patients is that the services provided are fully developed and their effectiveness has been established. For that reason, some clients/patients may not embrace the concept of research in practice settings, because conducting research implies uncertainty and the potential for risk. It is important that the reason for your study is clearly communicated and understood by all participants and that the study can be conducted with minimum interference with the provision of services. If your proposed study meets the standard definition of research on human subjects, it may need to be approved by an ethics committee in your organization, often called an institutional review board (IRB) or institutional ethics committee (IEC). All investigators—including students and practitioners—involved in human subjects research are generally required to take relevant online courses and be certified in the ethical and responsible conduct of human subjects research (Braunschweiger & Hansen, 2010). Many practitioner research studies do not require this kind of approval because they are focused more on institutional questions of evaluation. You need to ask your management or your instructor to find out more about the specific requirements in your setting.

Potential harms associated with practitioner research studies vary significantly. They most commonly include psychosocial stress, a sense of discomfort, and risks associated with revealing confidential personal information. Specific questions of disclosure are raised when withholding certain information from participants is part of the study's design so as to reduce certain biases. Intervention studies are designed explicitly to have specific effects on people and their environments and therefore need specific scrutiny in terms of unintended negative effects. You need to also consider risks associated with possible stigmatization, economic harms, and political ramifications. For example, collecting sociodemographic data from undocumented immigrants may put them at risk of losing their jobs or being deported.

Many ethical issues in practitioner research involve potential breaches of confidentiality. Therefore, practitioner researchers need to have robust procedures for safeguarding the privacy and confidentiality of the research data. Informed consent is also a central issue. IRB and IEC procedures emphasize the importance of obtaining informed consent—preferably in writing—prior to participants' involvement in a study. In obtaining informed consent you document the discussion of the research procedures with the participants, providing them the opportunity to ask questions and to obtain more information. If your study includes taking pictures or videos, you need to make your participants aware of such activities and obtain their written permission by way of photo/video release forms.

There is often confusion regarding the terms "privacy" and "confidentiality." They are not the same. Confidentiality is about acquiring sensitive information that your clients/patients share with you within a professional relationship for therapeutic, supportive, or educational purposes. Your clients/patients trust you to protect their confidential information and they expect you not to share such information with others; doing so would be considered a breach of confidentiality and, in most cases, a violation of professional ethics and regulations governing professional practice. The concept of privacy refers to each individual's rights to share or not share personal information related to their bodies, opinions, relationships, faith, and so on. The breach of privacy is when someone obtains access to a person's private information, observes or touches them inappropriately, or makes decisions for them without permission. In order to protect the privacy and confidentiality of clients/patients, practitioners need to follow the applicable rules and regulations, for example those of the Health Insurance Portability and Accountability Act (HIPAA) for accessing medical records and the Family Educational Rights and Privacy Act (FERPA) for student education records. Your management can provide information on which rules apply to your specific setting.

Logistical and Administrative Considerations

Consider how and where conversations related to your research are conducted. The places should be conducive to a comfortable exchange while providing the necessary privacy. Monetary or nonmonetary incentives can be provided as a token of appreciation for participants' time. It is always important to make every effort to accommodate individuals with disabilities or any types of medical or dietary restrictions (when, for example, providing refreshments for a focus group). Other administrative issues can include securing formal support from your management and supervisor, addressing any possible conflicts of interest, developing information materials tailored to the literacy level of the target audience, and having proactive procedures in place to address other problems inherent to conducting research, such as attrition or loss to follow-up.

Exercise 7. Ethical and Logistical Issues (see page 35)

1.8. Summary

In this chapter, the general concept of practitioner research was introduced. We learned about why we need practitioner research and discussed it in relation to other types of scientific investigation. Overall, practitioner research was described in terms of implementation science, other forms of research in health care and social services, and traditions close to the practitioner research approach. We learned that practitioner research is complementary to basic research and evaluation research in that they all facilitate the development of evidence-based practices, with practitioner research contributing specifically to the generation of valid and reliable practice-based evidence. In addition, we learned that as practitioners we engage in research—in collaboration with our colleagues, clients/patients, and other stakeholders—to improve our services. To do so, the importance of adopting an inquisitive mind-set was discussed, along with setting realistic expectations. The benefits of conducting practitioner research were described both at the practitioner and organizational levels. In general, practitioner research can enhance the level of learning and professional development among practitioners. It can help us make important decisions based on the local scientific evidence we generate through research and enhance our level of participation in improving our professional practices. This can ultimately lead to improving the quality of services and more effective use of new scientific discoveries in daily practice.

Practitioner research as described in this book is based on a framework consisting of the Practitioner Research Cycle and the Innovation Loop, comprised of seven key components. The key components were briefly discussed with illustrative examples, and the following chapters will be dedicated to one key component each. We learned that validity and reliability criteria in practitioner research are different than in other types of scientific inquiry, due primarily to the focus of practitioner research on solving practical problems within health care and social services settings. Such criteria include outcome validity, which is about whether the research was successful in solving the underlying practice problem and improving the practice. Another criterion is process validity (and its main domains; i.e., catalytic, democratic, and dialogical), which is described as a concept for assessing the robustness of the process with regard to the level of participation among the stakeholders and the iterative dynamics of engaging in practitioner research. By mapping those criteria to a hypothetical practitioner research study, we learned how to assess and improve the integrity of our research. Furthermore, several guidelines were introduced that could increase the validity and reliability of practitioner research. One important approach was through triangulation of sources of data, methods of data collection, and researchers. Moreover, we learned about five types of research questions that could be answered through practitioner research: descriptive, defining, comparative, evaluative, and explanatory. We also learned about the different levels on which practitioner research projects can be conducted: individual, departmental, organizational, interorganizational, and community.

The last section of this chapter was devoted to conducting practitioner research within the context of health care and social services settings. We learned how professional practice is set up primarily for providing effective services, which could pose significant challenges to the requirements of conducting robust research studies. Community, health care, and social services settings are each unique in terms of their needs and forms of functioning. A community is often formed around an identity that unites its members and defines its interactions. Resources and assets are usually shared through an informal web of social networks. And community members often act following ongoing debates and a collective wisdom. We learned that health care and social services settings are often set up according to hierarchical structures, each with unique disciplinary and cultural norms. Most importantly, it is critical not to view practitioner research as an add-on task, but rather as a way to improve practice in the interest of everyone involved: patients/clients, practitioners, organizations, and the professional fields of practice. Several strategies were discussed for becoming involved in practitioner research, generating support and resources, and creating more capacity for solving fundamental and often controversial problems. The principles of ethical and responsible conduct of research were discussed focusing on the privacy and confidentiality of the participants, the minimization of harm and potential risks, and maximization of the benefits found in being part of a research process.

Exercise 1. Practitioner Researchers' Dual Roles and Duty

When involved in practitioner research, you often find yourself wearing multiple hats that may lead to conflicts of interest. This is because, after all, you are a researcher, health or social work professional, and a member of your organization all at the same time. By doing this exercise, you will become more aware of these issues.

Meet with your colleagues and/or clients/patients as a group to discuss each of the following scenarios. For each scenario, identify potential conflicts of interest (given the multiple roles people play) and explore practical strategies to address them.

1. You have been commissioned to conduct a patient satisfaction survey for the purpose of showcasing your organization's exceptional customer service and state-of-the-art facilities. While you're doing your research, you notice that a colleague is not following the standard procedures of documenting and organizing his patients' counseling sessions.

2. You are going to a conference to present your research data. You believe that some of your negative findings, if they go public, could affect the image of your organization.

3. You are doing research to study the sexual feelings and experiences of patients with psychiatric issues. You need to interview several of your clients for whom you are their assigned counselor.

4. You have observed that the way some of your colleagues share information could be putting your clients at risk, but you cannot get the necessary funding to conduct a study to figure out how to best address the problem.

5. A colleague is calling in sick and asking you to cover his duties, but you have several important research activities planned for that day.

Exercise 2. Research Ownership

The ideal situation for conducting practitioner research is when the practitioner is fully interested in the topic and has developed a strong sense of ownership of the research. Sometimes, however, organizations don't follow this principle; they may ask you to conduct a study that you are not quite interested in or don't know much about. We have provided three examples. Set aside time and meet as a team with your colleagues to discuss your responses to the following hypothetical requests from management and explore different possible ways for addressing the issues presented.

1. Management is interested in better use of the office space. They ask you to conduct research on this topic and give them a report.

2. The board members of your organization have been working with management on a research plan for several months. The design is now complete and they ask you to conduct the study.

3. The organization has developed a set of quality control measures and indicators that you believe are incomplete and unsatisfactory. However, they insist that you conduct a study based on those metrics.

Exercise 3. The Stages of the Practitioner Research Method

A practitioner's disciplinary background (e.g., health care, social work, psychology, nursing) influences his or her perspective on practitioner research. This exercise will help you develop an understanding for practitioner research based on your professional training and experience.

Think about a new approach that was implemented in your professional practice. Now, review the key components of the Practitioner Research Method and consider if defining and implementing the approach reflects the stages of practitioner research. The goal is to determine to what extent information was gathered and analyzed in the development of the initiative. Think about ways in which the adoption of the approach could have been more strongly grounded in practice-based evidence. You may want to ask your colleagues to join you in this exercise so you can explore the possibility of using your own research to further develop your professional practice, considering the costs and benefits of doing so.

Exercise 4. Triangulation

Imagine that you are working on a practitioner research assignment to improve the effectiveness and quality of team meetings in your organization. This study is presumably designed to identify current procedures and processes for scheduling, setting agendas, facilitating discussions, documenting results, and following up on the decisions.

Either individually or as a group, identify a diverse group of practitioners to form a research team to work on this topic. Consider how to generate valid and reliable results based on the triangulation of sources, methods, and researchers.

Exercise 5. Types of Research Questions

A physical therapist notices that there are ambiguities with regard to the diagnosis and treatment of impaired movement in patients with chronic lower back pain at her clinic. She wants to understand the problem by first exploring ideas from more experienced colleagues and by reviewing the published professional and research literature for the purpose of identifying the most current recommendations. In addition, she wants to review the medical records for former patients in order to describe the underlying causes, signs and symptoms, and treatment protocols. She suspects that older patients with herniated disks are less likely to receive the type of treatment they need. If she's correct, it may be possible to design and test a specific standard operating procedure for this kind of patient. She's also interested in conducting an overall evaluation of the organization's procedures for managing lower back pain.

Based on the above scenario, draft an example for each of the five types of research questions that the physical therapist could use in her study (descriptive, defining, comparative, evaluative, explanatory).

Ask two other colleagues to do the same, share your notes, and reflect on each other's questions.

Finally, discuss potential research designs for answering each type of research question.

Exercise 6. Research Context of Your Organization

After learning about the special characteristics of health care and social services settings, it's time to examine research in the context of your own organization. To do so, list four important practice problems that you want to solve and write them down in the following table. For each practice problem, identify its type, whether it is a pragmatic problem (i.e., less controversial daily issues with a larger appeal) or a strategic problem (i.e., requiring controversial changes in policy and institutional culture). In addition, for each problem, identify potential enabling factors; challenges and limitations you might face; and any expected benefits for the practitioners, clients/patients, and organization once the problem is solved.

Practice problem	Type of problem	Enabling factors	Challenges and limitations	Expected benefits

Exercise 7. Ethical and Logistical Issues

Use the same practice problems that you identified in Exercise 6 and propose hypothetical practitioner research studies (e.g., conducting a survey, designing an instrument, organizing a training) to address each problem. For each proposed practitioner research study, write down potential risks and benefits for your clients/patients and any logistical arrangements and approvals—for example, from an institutional review board or independent ethics committee—that you would need to secure before conducting the study.

Practitioner research	Potential risks	Benefits to the clients	Logistical arrangements	Needed approvals

REFERENCES

Anderson, G. L., Herr, K., & Nihlen, A. S. (2007). *Studying your own school: An educator's guide to practitioner action research*. Corwin Press.

Altrichter, H., Feldman, A., Posch, P., & Somekh, B. (2008). *Teachers investigate their work: An introduction to action research across the profession*. Routledge.

Balas, E. A., & Boren, S. A. (2000). Managing clinical knowledge for health care improvement. *Yearbook of Medical Informatics*, *1*, 65–70.

Bania, M., & Roebuck, B. (2018). *Local adaptations of crime prevention programs: Finding the optimal balance between fidelity and fit*. Research Report 2017-R019-A. Public Safety Canada.

BBC History. (2014). Sigmund Freud (1856–1939). http://www.bbc.co.uk/history/historic_figures/freud_sigmund.shtml

Bero, L. A., Grilli, R., Grimshaw, J. M., Harvey, E., Oxman, A. D., & Thomson, M. A. (1998). Closing the gap between research and practice: an overview of systematic reviews of interventions to promote the implementation of research findings. The Cochrane Effective Practice and Organization of Care Review Group. *BMJ (Clinical Research Ed.)*, *317*(7156), 465–468.

Braunschweiger, P., & Hansen, K. (2010). Collaborative institutional training initiative (CITI). *Journal of Clinical Research Best Practices*, *6*(4), 1–6.

Brownson, R. C. (2012). *Dissemination and implementation research in health: Translating science to practice* (1st ed.). Oxford University Press.

Brownson, R. C. (2017). *Dissemination and implementation research in health: Translating science to practice* (2nd ed.). Oxford University Press.

Bryman, A. (2004). Triangulation and measurement. In M. S. Lewis-Beck, A. Bryman, & T. Futing Liao (Eds.), *Encyclopedia of Social Science Research Methods* (pp. 1143–1144). Sage.

Bolhuis, S. (2012). Praktijkonderzoek als professionele leerstrategie in onderwijs en opleiding [Practitioner research as a professional learning strategy in education and training]. In S. Bolhuis & Q. Kools (Eds.), *Praktijkonderzoek als professionele leerstrategie in onderwijs en opleiding* [Practitioner research as a professional learning strategy in education and training] (pp. 15–44). Fontys Lerarenopleiding.

Centers for Disease Control and Prevention (CDC). (n.d.). *Understanding evidence: Evidence based decision-making summary.* Retrieved March 1, 2021. https://vetoviolence.cdc.gov/apps/evidence/docs/EBDM_82412.pdf

Cooper, P. A. (1993). Paradigm shifts in designed instruction: From behaviorism to cognitivism to constructivism. *Educational Technology*, *33*(5), 12–19.

Damschroder, L. J., Aron, D. C., Keith, R. E., Kirsh, S. R., Alexander, J. A., & Lowery, J. C. (2009). Fostering implementation of health services research findings into practice: A consolidated framework for advancing implementation science. *Implementation Science*, *4*(1), 50.

Durlak, J. A., & DuPre, E. P. (2008). Implementation matters: A review of research on the influence of implementation on program outcomes and the factors affecting implementation. *American Journal of Community Psychology*, *41*(3–4), 327.

Gabbay, J., & le May, A. (2016). Mindlines: Making sense of evidence in practice. *British Journal of General Practice*, *66*(649), 402–403. https://www.ncbi.nlm.nih.gov/pmc/articles/PMC4979949

George, A. L. (2019). Case studies and theory development: The method of structured, focused comparison. In *Alexander L. George: A pioneer in political and social sciences* (pp. 191–214). Springer.

Green, L. W. (2006). Public health asks of systems science: To advance our evidence-based practice, can you help us get more practice-based evidence? *American Journal of Public Health*, *96*(3), 406–409.

Glasgow, R. E., Lichtenstein, E., & Marcus, A. C. (2003). Why don't we see more translation of health promotion research to practice? Rethinking the efficacy-to-effectiveness transition. *American Journal of Public Health*, *93*(8), 1261–1267.

Golafshani, N. (2003). Understanding reliability and validity in qualitative research. *The Qualitative Report*, *8*(4), 597–606.

Harinck, F. (2007). *Basisprincipes praktijkonderzoek* [Basic principles of practitioner research]. Garant.

Heiner, M. (1988). *Praxisforschung in der sozialen Arbeit* [Practitioner research in social work]. Lambertus-Verlag.

Herr, K., & Anderson, G. L. (2015). *The action research dissertation: A guide for students and faculty* (2nd ed.). Sage.

ICPHR (International Collaboration for Participatory Health Research). (2013). *Position paper 1: What is participatory health research?* http://www.icphr.org/uploads/2/0/3/9/20399575/ichpr_position_paper_1_defintion_-_version_may_2013.pdf

Israel, B. A., Schulz, A. J., Parker, E. A., & Becker, A. B. (1998). Review of community-based research: Assessing partnership approaches to improve public health. *Annual Review of Public Health*, *19*(1), 173–202.

Kilo, C. M. (1998). A framework for collaborative improvement: Lessons from the Institute for Healthcare Improvement's Breakthrough Series. *Quality Management in Health Care*, *6*(4), 1–14.

Kolb, D. A. (1984). *Experiential learning.* Prentice Hall.

Lee, A. S. (1991). Integrating positivist and interpretive approaches to organizational research. *Organization Science*, *2*(4), 342–365.

Maykus, S. (2010). *Praxisforschung in der Kinder- und Jugendhilfe: Theorie, Beispiele und Entwicklungsoptionen eines Forschungsfeldes* [Practice research in children and youth services: Theory, examples, and the potential for further development]. VS-Verlag.

Moser, C. O. (1989). Gender planning in the Third World: Meeting practical and strategic gender needs. *World Development, 17*(11), 1799–1825.

Reason, P., & Bradbury, H. (Eds.). (2001). *Handbook of action research: Participative inquiry and practice.* Sage.

Rogers, E. M., & Shoemaker, F. F. (1971). *Communication of innovations: A cross-cultural approach.* Free Press.

Sackett, D. L. (1997, February). Evidence-based medicine. *Seminars in Perinatology 21*(1), 3–5).

Smeijsters, H., et al. (2011). *Kenmerken, randvoorwaarden en criteria van praktijkgericht zorgonderzoek* [Features, requirements, and criteria of practice-based research in health care]. HBORaad, Zon MW.

Smith, L. S., & Wilkins, N. (2018). Mind the gap: Approaches to addressing the research-to-practice, practice-to-research chasm. *Journal of Public Health Management and Practice, 24*(Suppl 1), S6.

Starman, A. B. (2013). The case study as a type of qualitative research. *Journal of Contemporary Educational Studies / Sodobna Pedagogika, 64*(1).

Van der Donk, C., & Van Lanen, B. (2019). *Praktijkonderzoek in zorg en welzijn* [Practitioner research in health care and social work] (3rd ed.). Uitgeverij Coutinho.

Van der Donk, C., & Van Lanen, B. (2020). *Praktijkonderzoek in de school* [Practitioner research in education] (4th ed.). Uitgeverij Coutinho.

Van der Donk, C., Van Lanen, B., & Wright, M. T. (2014). *Praxisforschung im Sozial- und Gesundheitswesen* [Practitioner research in social work and health care]. Hogrefe Verlag / Verlag Hans Huber.

Van den Akker, J. (1999). Principles and methods of development research. In J. van den Akker, R. M. Branch, K. Gustafson, N. Nieveen, & T. Plomp (Eds.), *Design approaches and tools in education and training* (pp. 1–14). Kluwer Academic. https://doi.org/10.1007/978-94-011-4255-7

Van Keken, H. (2006). *Voor het onderzoek: Het formuleren van een probleemstelling* [Starting research: Formulating a problem definition]. Boom onderwijs.

Webb, E. J., Campbell, D. T., Schwartz, R. D., & Sechrest, L. (1966). *Unobtrusive measures: Nonreactive measures in the social sciences.* Rand McNally.

Van Vliet, K. (2009). *Nieuwe eisen aan de sociale professionals: De wisselwerking tussen competentieontwikkeling en kennisontwikkeling* [New demands for social work professionals: The interaction between competence development and knowledge development]. Verwey-Jonker Instituut.

Wenger, E. (1998). Communities of practice: Learning as a social system. *Systems Thinker, 9*(5), 2–3.

Westfall, J. M., Mold, J., & Fagnan, L. (2007). Practice-based research—"Blue Highways" on the NIH roadmap. *JAMA, 297*(4), 403–406.

Wright, M.T. (2013). Was ist Partizipative Gesundheitsforschung? [What is Participatory Health Research? Position paper of the International Collaboration for Participatory Health Research]. *Prävention und Gesundheitsförderung, 8*(3), 122–131.

Zerhouni, E. (2003). The NIH roadmap. *Science, 302*(5642), 63–72. https://doi.org/10.1126/science.1091867

2

Orientation

There are a few questions to answer when you first contemplate conducting practitioner research, starting with the issue of concern that you want to address (figure 2.1). How is it defined? What is the scope of the problem? What do you expect to learn in terms of how to improve your practice? Do you need to conduct research to address the problem or are there other options? It is best to discuss these questions in practice with other professionals so you can collectively gain a deeper understanding of what practitioner research can bring to you and your organization as well as generate clarity, consensus, energy, and enthusiasm.

In this chapter, first we discuss common reasons that some practitioners are interested in conducting research and then explain several techniques that a practitioner could use to identify significant practice problems. Once a practice problem is identified, explorative problem analysis is used to explore the issue from multiple perspectives. The result will be a detailed description of the practice problem defined in a way that could be used to determine the research focus (the next key component of the Practitioner Research Method that is fully discussed in chapter 3). This chapter, in the meantime, concludes with a summary of takeaways and relevant exercises.

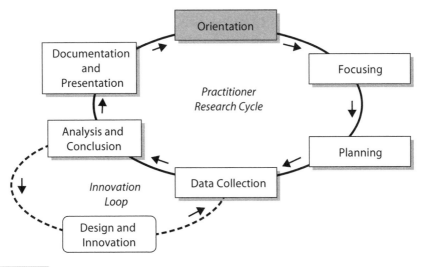

Figure 2.1

Key component of practitioner research: Orientation

2.1. Common Reasons to Conduct Practitioner Research

There are many reasons practitioners become interested in research. Some of the most common ones are described here.

Personal and Professional

Sometimes there are situations in practice settings that require careful examination and exploration. Imagine that you are working in a clinic where a specific treatment is not working as expected and does not result in the desired outcomes. Or perhaps your clients are complaining about the quality of services, or they say that your reception area is not quite welcoming. You may find yourself interested in doing something about one of these problems, but you realize that you need to gain more insights and collect research data to do so.

Practitioners often have great ideas about why the problems occur and how they can be fixed. These ideas usually stem from repeated observations, anecdotal accounts, and in-depth discussions with colleagues and management. Research can help you collect the empirical data you need to test your hypothesis. Most practitioners, once immersed in research, find themselves on a never-ending trajectory of discovery and impact.

Institutional

There are often pressing issues and practice problems leading to a collective desire for conducting research at the institutional level. In some cases, the management encourages empirical research to gain better insights about the problems so they can be handled more effectively. As a result, research is often highly encouraged and even required in such institutions. Some examples include encouraging staff to study or learn how to assess their professional needs and act more effectively, a quality report pointing out the need for a more in-depth research study, practitioner research being aligned with an existing policy (e.g., client safety being part of a memorandum of understanding with partners), or new national programs requiring local implementation and evaluation.

External

Opportunities for conducting practitioner research may arise from programs first conducted by other organizations. For example, an educational institution may launch a study to strengthen the social network of elderly people residing in assisted-living contexts. They may choose to institute an intergenerational neighborhood program with health education, screening, and consultation components. This kind of program can create opportunities for practitioners' engagement in research studies that are beneficial to all parties involved.

These overarching motives indicate that people choose to engage in practitioner research for varied reasons. And even as research in a practice setting can be initiated and conducted at different levels (e.g., providers, management, other institutions), it usually focuses on the same level from which the research concept is originated. For example, management is concerned about management issues and frontline staff are concerned with issues related to patient or client contact. Focusing on a topic related to your area of responsibility fosters a sense of ownership and grassroots leadership needed to implement the study and disseminate the findings. In chapter 1 we discussed how research and professional practice are inherently intertwined. Health care and social work professionals are expected to engage in practitioner research to pursue the goals and objectives of their own professional practice. Therefore, practitioner research can be viewed as a professional learning strategy. It's important that you find personal and educational value in conducting research.

> *Example.* The following quote, taken from a research plan, is from a practitioner researcher who describes why they are interested in conducting research at a senior center:
>
>> I work in a senior residential care center where I joined a working group to improve the quality of services provided to the residents. After reviewing the literature and studying the current practices related to our topic, we noted a lack of sensitivity to the needs of gay residents. For example, we found out that almost half of the caregivers assumed that the home has few or no homosexuals. Therefore, we requested this to be our research project. Personally, I would like to determine which measures the home can take to better accommodate our elderly homosexual patients. I intend to present the results to all staff in a dedicated meeting. It's because I have been concerned for a long time with the lack of sexual diversity in our care system. I became aware that I do not sufficiently appreciate the fact that some patients might have a different sexual orientation. I feel this affects their sense of well-being and the quality of care that they receive. I hope my research enables me to provide better care to our elderly gay patients.

For practitioner research studies commissioned by a third party, you need to develop a good understanding of why the study is being requested. Keep in mind that sometimes your reason for doing the research may be different from that of the other parties. This can lead to some challenging dilemmas and they need to be handled with care. In the next example, a child and youth care facility only allows outdoor materials to be developed, while the practitioner is more interested in better understanding items that could be used both indoors and outdoors:

> *Example.* When it's come to serving the needs of severely disabled children, I wish to develop excellent materials for indoor and outdoor playing and learning activities. The materials for our indoor use are outdated and we hardly have any toys or games for outdoor activities. This research could be an excellent opportunity for gaining a deeper knowledge about ways of better stimulating play activities among these children. But the coordinator of the facility where I work insists that we should only develop materials for outdoor use. She believes that nothing is wrong with the indoor toys and games.

It's very important to discuss and resolve these conflicting opinions earlier in the process.

A practitioner research project usually starts with a vague problem, not a clearly defined research question. In this book, we use the umbrella term "practice problem" to refer to all situations arising in professional practice that may become a starting point for in-depth studies. It is used broadly to refer to challenges, opportunities, needs, and areas that can be improved. Therefore, it is important not to misinterpret the term as meaning only problematic situations. Practice problems can be classified in the following categories:

- Real-life situations in which you may not be quite confident how they need to be handled (uncertainty)
- Challenging dilemmas that need robust and clear answers (challenges)
- The need to improve the effectiveness and/or quality of services or develop new components for the organization (enhancement)
- Desired learning outcomes of providers, experts, management teams, etc. (learning)
- Making sure that we are doing the right thing (validation)
- Anticipating future developments (anticipation)
- Sustaining resources by satisfying funding agencies' expectations (sustainability)
- Introducing best practices and contributing to professional practice (dissemination and scalability)

Sometimes these categories overlap. Following are examples of practice problems that could be the focus of research:

- High incidence of bullying among students
- Addressing health disparities among minorities by enhancing cultural competency
- Establishing rapport with homeless adolescents
- Strengthening social cohesion among a group of 12- to 21-year-old mental health patients with behavioral problems
- Inadequacy of aftercare for alcohol-addicted youth
- Motivating senior colleagues to attend peer coaching sessions
- Improving patient safety through better understanding of reporting and registration processes

As discussed, some practice problems arise from real-life experiences. For instance, a few girls participating in a life-skills training program may not be able to practice some of the skills to the same extent as the other participants. This situation can generate several questions: Which skills are most challenging and why? Why those specific girls? What do they have in common? What does the training program offer?

In some scenarios, practice problems are presented for their potential to generate "solutions" or to "innovate" new practical interventions. In this case, you need to step back for a moment and ask yourself, "Why do I want to improve the situation? What are the underlying benefits associated with the desired innovation?" The answers to these questions not only prepare and motivate you for the task, but they guide you throughout the process, so you know what you are supposed to achieve.

However, not all practice problems are equally suited to be the subject of practitioner research. You need to put the tasks in perspective. Sometimes, you may not have enough time or resources to find answers to certain research questions. Your first challenge is to identify a practice problem that both you and other members of your team are interested in exploring. You will gain more internal support if the research adds value for others in the field. It allows you to benefit more from the expertise and experience of your colleagues as well.

> *Example.* Judith is required for her graduation to conduct practitioner research and she is free to choose her topic of interest. During her internship at the youth center, she noticed a downward trend in youth participation in the center's activities. This issue has been frequently mentioned at the center's internal meetings as well. Judith offered to write a research plan on this issue and asked the board for approval. Her proposal is well received, and the board appointed a project team to support her.

This example also shows how Judith became inspired and defined her practice problem by talking with and listening to her colleagues.

Here we describe six techniques through which you could systematically discover practice problems within your organization: brainstorming, keeping a journal, reflection, observation, and dialogue.

Technique 1: Brainstorming

Brainstorming is an associative technique, which means it intrigues you and others to generate ideas, information, and insights associated with keywords in a simple question. This technique helps generate a wealth of knowledge and experience rooted in the topic of interest. For example, through brainstorming you can generate useful statements, past events, questions, and previous problems or incidents related to your professional practice. Some common guiding questions in a brainstorming session are:

- What are some of the issues that we are facing?
- During the past week, what questions and problems have been discussed?
- What are some of the situations that we are not handling very well?
- Which aspects of the organization negatively affect our ability to communicate effectively?
- What are some of the specific aspects of our professional care that should be improved?
- What are our greatest strengths and weaknesses from our colleagues' perspectives?

You can brainstorm on your own, but it works best in a group because you can use the associations of other group members and tap into their collective wisdom. One important rule for brainstorming is to write everything down that comes to your mind without filtering your thoughts. You can group your thoughts in clusters of related words to stimulate the process. In a group setting, encourage everyone to participate freely and discourage criticizing other team members' comments. You can end the process by reviewing the output and putting a checkmark next to a statement that indicates a potential practice problem. Lastly, you may want to look for recurring topics and any correlating themes. Group brainstorming can lead to broader overall support for your project.

Technique 2: Keeping a Journal

Writing notes in a journal is a good way to keep track of your best ideas and daily experiences. You may choose to log the events as they occur or make entries at the end of the day. Many interesting experiences and thoughts can be documented in your journal. But first you need to decide how you want to document them and how to use the information. You may choose to review some relevant articles and add the information to your journal. This can help you identify your practice problem by learning from other research studies while making your own observations. It is always a good idea to review your journal entries at the end of a set period, such as one week. The purpose is to mark important themes and try to identify one or more practice problems based on your journal's information. An example with entries and notes is illustrated in table 2.1.

If possible, you can ask your colleagues or clients/patients to keep their own journals, too, so you can share your information with each other and agree upon common practice problems. But this will depend on the level of the intervention. For example, you may suggest that management and frontline staff keep journals if the purpose of your practitioner research is to improve the overall performance of the institution. However, if you are solely interested in assessing and improving your own services, a personal journal is sufficient and can later be supplemented with input from your clients/patients and colleagues.

Table 2.1 Example of journal entries from a physical therapist		
Day	Log	Main issues and questions
Tuesday	*During physical therapy* Tim indicates that last week he was in a lot of pain during his exercises. I asked him to demonstrate how he performs the exercises. It turned out he did not follow my instructions properly and he was putting too much strain on his back. Tim says he found my instructions somewhat unclear. He would have preferred an illustrated step-by-step guide.	What are my options if instructions are not followed properly? How can we explain the exercises more clearly in our brochure?
Wednesday	*During session* I was called in to help Mrs. Fleet, who had hip surgery, with her physical exercise. Our training focuses on teaching Mrs. Fleet how to move around with a walker. She expressed that her home environment is vastly different from the hospital, which creates a challenge about what type of movement is relevant and feasible for her. I demonstrate the proper way to walk, sit, lie down, and get up. In addition, Mrs. Fleet has hearing difficulties that affect our communications. She has trouble hearing most of what I say.	Contrast between hospital and home environment. How can we better accommodate patients with hearing difficulties?

Technique 3: Developing a Self-Reflective Report

Reflecting is about reviewing how well you and your colleagues are functioning in your job at both the individual level and as a team. Reflecting helps you to understand new ways for improving your performance.

A self-reflective report is where you document the process and the results of your reflection on that process. A well-written report can be a useful source of insights and information needed for both identifying and exploring practice problems. A good reflective report contains the following elements (Geenen, 2017):

- What prompted your reflection (starting point/objectives)?
- What is your conclusion (ending point/outcome)?
- What facts led to the conclusion? What helped and what didn't?
- What is the significance of your conclusion?
- What are some of the views about your actions, thoughts, and ideas that would qualify as new results?

Review your reflective report thoroughly and mark passages that you find interesting. In a second review, write down new questions and issues that come to mind. Be attentive of patterns and associations that could be useful to clarify your practice problem. Like brainstorming and journaling techniques, reflective reports can be a source of inspiration backed by comments from your clients/patients and colleagues.

Technique 4: Being Observed by a Client/Patient or Colleague

This technique is simply about asking a colleague or a client/patient to observe your work and provide you with feedback. It would be helpful to create a chart or a checklist of items needed to be observed and discussed (more details are provided in chapter 5). Then you ask the observer to mark or write down statements about your performance. Through discussing the observation results with your observer, you may come across patterns that could inform potential practice problems. The unique strength of this technique lies in its ability to bring certain behaviors and actions to your attention that otherwise could be missed.

Technique 5: Having Short Conversations with Colleagues, Clients/Patients, and Others

Short, ad hoc conversations can be a good source of information. Talking with others who have different roles or experiences is always a good strategy to learn more about problems and issues. But first you need to be selective about who you choose for your conversations. It could be someone in a leadership position, a practitioner with more experience than you, or a client/patient who is receiving services. Second, you need to spend some time assembling a set of relevant questions to ask and to prepare for the discussion. During the conversation, you can use the brainstorming questions and techniques to enrich your conversation. Some natural opportunities for short conversations are during lunchtime, before or after a session with a client/patient, in the visitors' area, or in a staff room. Lastly, you need to write down a summary of the main points as soon as possible. Like other techniques, look for patterns in your notes that could inform an interesting practice problem.

Technique 6: Reviewing Internal Sources

Internal sources can help you identify current practice problems within your organization when observing the following steps:

- Take note of important results evaluations, annual reports, and other assessments involving colleagues or other stakeholders.
- Review relevant meeting notes and records of special events and trainings.
- Review any available self-assessment forms, individual development plans, and institutional policy documents.
- Read the news and announcements posted on the organization's website and social media.

Exercise 1. Identifying Suitable Practice Problems (see page 62)

2.3. Mapping the Context of Professional Practice

Mapping can be referred to as a context analysis of professional practice based on your own observations, experiences, conversations with colleagues, and review of relevant sources. The outcome of a context analysis can help you identify your practice problem, select an appropriate design for your practitioner research project, and determine the communication and reporting strategies that you would use after conducting the project. The following section describes a procedure for analyzing and mapping the context of the professional practice where you intend to conduct your project and provides a useful overview of relevant needs, assets, and programs that you should include.

Characteristics of Professional Practice

Describe the professional context where the research will take place. Discuss specific characteristics of professional practice relevant to your research project using the following checklist and answering those questions relevant to your project. Add more questions, if needed.

Mission, vision, core values, and policy of the organization: What are they? What are the stated goals and strategic objectives of the organization? What does this mean for the daily work of the practitioners?

External environment: What significant demographic, economic, cultural, technological, ecological, and sociopolitical transitions and changes are happening in the external environment? What changes are relevant to your project?

Organizational structure: What does the organizational structure look like?

Table 2.2. Examples of relevant current developments within a health care organization	
Level	Issues, initiatives, research projects, and innovations
Individual	During client contact the emphasis is mainly on promoting self-regulation.
Departmental	Since the beginning of 2019 multidisciplinary consultation has taken place weekly. Many staff members have recently enrolled in a training course on patient engagement.
Organizational	Promoting client participation is one of the main goals of the organization. Recently a research study was conducted about the privacy of clients and data-sharing practices.
Interorganizational	A new collaboration has started with another health care organization to explore the possibilities for staff exchange.
Community	As a result of changing policy at the state level, providers need to more explicitly document the impact of their services and share them with other stakeholders.

Primary process: How are the primary work processes organized and flowing? Who are the clients? Where are the clients mostly located? How does the organization interact and serve its clients?

Quality management: What quality management system is in place? Who are the key players? How does the system work?

Organizational culture: How would you characterize the organizational culture?

Interests: Are there any special interests, conflicts of interest, tensions, or differences of opinion that you should take into account?

Daily dynamics: How do you characterize the daily routine?

Language use: Which terms and abbreviations are used in the organization that can be unclear to outsiders?

Preconditions: What are some of the mandatory procedures, guidelines, and standards that need to be followed? Are the requirements of your project, such as the availability of frontline staff and spaces, in place?

Relevant Current Developments

Provide an overview of issues and initiatives that are—or recently have been—the focus of attention in the organization at different levels (e.g., individual, departmental, organizational). Also describe what research projects and innovations have recently been carried out in the organization. An example is provided in table 2.2.

2.4. Selecting a Practice Problem

At this stage, you should have generated ideas about a few promising practice problems. To make an informed decision, however, you need to create a set of criteria that your practice problem must meet to qualify. A good practice problem scores relatively high in most criteria, with fewer low scores compared to the other candidates. You may want to share your criteria with your colleagues and ask them to help you decide. Remember, the more people you have who approve your choice, the broader support you will gain for your research.

Here are some examples of common criteria used by practitioner researchers:

Related to your own professional development

- I have a keen interest in this practice problem.

- It is a priority for me that I address this practice problem.

- Exploring this practice problem helps me learn and grow professionally so I can become a better practitioner.

- Studying this practice problem is beneficial to me in the following ways . . .

Related to the organization

- This practice problem concerns many of my colleagues.

- Solving this practice problem could improve the quality of our services.

- It is a priority for the organization that I address this practice problem.

- The organization's knowledge and understanding of this practice problem is low.

- Studying this practice problem is beneficial to the organization in the following ways . . .

Related to professional practice in general and to society

- This practice problem is socially relevant.

- This problem relates to developments in the professional field.

- This problem has been identified by professionals outside of my organization.

- Studying this practice problem is beneficial to the profession and society in the following ways . . .

Related to the practicality and logistics of the project

- Practitioner research seems to be an appropriate strategy to tackle this practice problem.

- My position in the organization enables me to address this practice problem.

If you are expected to conduct practitioner research as part of your training, make sure that you comply with your professional code of ethics (as discussed in the previous chapter) and your institution's internal policies and requirements.

Exercise 2. Create Your Own Set of Criteria (see page 62)

2.5. Exploratory Problem Analysis

At this stage, you know why you are interested in conducting your practitioner research and you have selected a relevant practice problem. Now you can start your exploratory problem analysis. Bear in mind that it's likely that you'll need to adjust and change your research proposal based on new insights and information that you gain.

It's even possible that you will realize that your original practice problem is not the real issue, and you will need to replace it with something else.

Example. You notice some negative interactions among a group of 12–14 adolescents in an after-school program. In a meeting with your colleagues, they validate your observation and encourage you to explore the social behavior of that group as your practice problem. You like the idea, but you decide to further explore their interactions before finishing your research proposal. So, you start talking with a few of the students and their parents. Meanwhile, you keep a journal and document your experiences. The results lead you to the conclusion that tension in the group is caused by transitioning from middle school to high school rather than being a behavioral problem. Therefore, you decide to revise your work and explore the issue of transitioning.

There are nine techniques for conducting an exploratory analysis of your practice problem. These techniques help you better understand the factors that are associated with your practice problem and some of its possible root causes. In doing so, we try to show you ways to integrate your and your colleagues' perspectives on how the practice problem is conceptualized. The analysis helps you become more oriented to the problem and its scope through acquisition of valuable information. At the beginning, you may think that the process takes lots of time, but soon you will notice the value of your investment and be rewarded with great returns, such as a better description of your practice problem and a better sense of how to conduct your exploratory problem analysis and literature review.

The first four techniques are based on associative reasoning, helping you and your colleagues to generate a set of associative responses to provide a full coverage of different aspects of your practice problem. The other five techniques focus on exploring the practice problem from different perspectives to deepen your understanding of it.

Technique 1: Brainstorming on the Practice Problem

The same brainstorming technique discussed earlier can be used to explore different aspects of the problem and its associated factors. For example, if you are exploring the practice problem of "patients' satisfaction with occupational therapy sessions," you could ask the following brainstorming questions: What are the sociodemographic characteristics of the patients who are utilizing the services? What are some of the strengths and weaknesses of the therapies related to the patient population?

Technique 2: Mind Mapping

The mind-mapping technique was developed by Tony Buzan in 2003. In this process an organizational (tree) chart is used to connect different aspects of the practice problem and create a more holistic view of the situation. In this approach, sub-themes branch out from the stem, where your practice problem is located, like a tree. The mind-mapping process enables you to make connections between fragments of information and create a big picture of the problem.

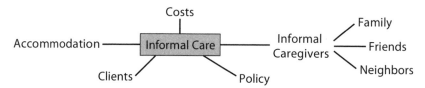

Figure 2.2

Excerpt from a mind map on informal care

Having a detailed visualization of the knowledge and ideas regarding your key concept is a great starting point for communicating with others. In addition, this will validate your previous knowledge, deepen your understanding, and help you build consensus. You may be surprised to learn that your original assessment of the problem was incomplete or incorrect. You may also learn that there are many differences of opinion in your organization about the nature of the problem and how it should be handled. Therefore, it would be enlightening to merge different mind maps and analyze them. You will see how people can make critical contributions simply because their styles of thinking are different. Asking others to provide their associative responses will give you a multifaceted view of the practice problem.

You may conduct your own mind-mapping session using one of the following three strategies: (1) build your own mind map first, share it with others, and incorporate their associative responses into the map; (2) in a group setting, draw your own mind maps individually, share and reflect on each other's maps, and get inspired to draw a group map; or (3) develop one common mind map as a group. A mind map on aspects of informal care is illustrated in figure 2.2.

Drawing a Mind Map

1. Define a main theme for your practice problem that could be placed at the center of your mind map.
2. Find and connect relevant key concepts to your main theme, which would become your larger branches.
3. Find and attach relevant sub-themes to their respective concepts to form the smaller branches. You may continue this process and subdivide the small branches, if desired.
4. Draw on theoretical knowledge to expand your mind map. If one mind map is not enough, you may want to create other mind maps.

Technique 3: Concept Mapping

Concept maps are similar to mind maps, but they often provide more complex visual illustrations of hierarchical structures and dynamic processes. They usually entail some interrelationships between the themes and sub-themes. If well executed, concept mapping can illustrate the practice problem clearly and serve as a guide for the development of the research plan. Some concept maps show the flow of activities in a logical order and are often called either *flowcharts* or *logic models* (figure 2.3). On the other hand, some concept maps have hierarchical structures to depict different ecological levels and their interrelationships (figure 2.4). Lastly, *mixed-concept maps* will have both qualities, and are often used to simplify complex phenomena or theoretical models (figure 2.5). Unlike mind maps, concept maps often have more than one central theme.

Developing a Concept Map

You can develop your concept map by starting with a mind-mapping exercise.

1. Write down all associative responses related to your practice problem.
2. Prioritize your responses according to their importance; list the key concepts and add their associated sub-themes.
3. Where possible, arrange the key concepts either logically (sequentially) or hierarchically to form a network structure without one centralized nucleus.
4. Connect related domains and constructs with either a line or an arrow. Define the relationships with relevant verbs or nouns, if desired.
5. Consolidate your concept map by incorporating relevant theoretical models. Create a second concept map if one is not enough.

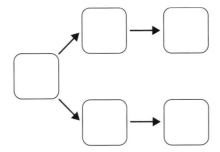

Figure 2.3

Example of a concept map with a logical structure

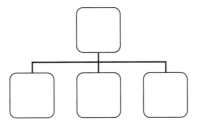

Figure 2.4

Example of a concept map with a hierarchical structure

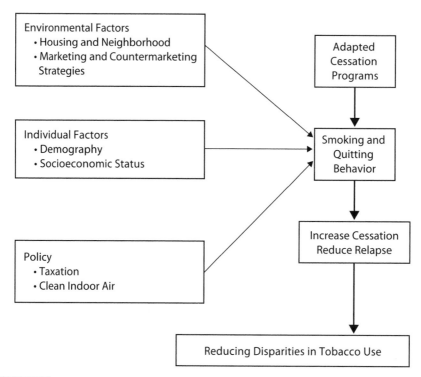

Figure 2.5

Example of a mixed-concept map for reducing disparities in tobacco use

Technique 4: Freewriting

Freewriting is defined as a technique through which one writes continuously and un-interrupted without being concerned about the grammar or the logical flow of statements. Some authors refer to this as a prewriting technique, as it produces raw material that can later be revised. Freewriting is another associative technique that can help you explore uncharted territories and make discoveries about your subconscious ideas and experiences regarding the practice problem. It can be done individually or with your colleagues and/or clients/patients. Keep in mind that this method will generate a substantial amount of raw material that can be revised or changed. But if done correctly, you can access some unexpected insights that could otherwise be overlooked.

Applying Freewriting

1. Start by describing the practice problem in a few lines using your own words.

2. Before beginning the actual freewriting, contemplate the practice problem for a few minutes to collect your thoughts.

3. Set a timer for 3–10 minutes and start writing continuously about the practice problem.

4. Write down anything that comes to your mind without being concerned about the grammar, punctuation, or writing style.

5. Review your notes and mark the statements that contain any valuable information.

6. In a group, ask everyone to mark their important statements, generate a combined list, and make sure that you keep track of who wrote what statements.

7. Identify patterns and connections between statements that are associated with the practice problem.

Technique 5: Review of the Literature

Reviewing scientific peer-reviewed and professional literature can help you gain a better understanding of the practice problem and its associated factors. First, you need to identify materials from different sources on topics related to your practice problem. Authors with different disciplinary perspectives often approach the practice problem differently with distinct terminologies. This can enhance your ability to deconstruct and recompose the issue in a way that works best for you. Good literature reviews often culminate in an overview of the common theories, background, and historical scientific enquiries related to your practice problem. They can also provide you with food for thought around the gaps in the literature by illuminating areas that we still don't know enough about (see appendix for more information). This information will help you stay relevant and guide you through the stages of your exploratory research. More specifically, a good literature review will provide you with a solid foundation for moving on to the next key component of the practitioner research, which is "Focusing." At this stage, you are trying to identify a few key sources to help you deepen your understanding of the practice problem. The literature review will be expanded as you develop your research project further (chapter 3).

> *Example.* Elizabeth and Stacy are both student interns working in a foster care organization. Members of the organization expressed a need for a special training to enhance cooperation between biological and foster parents. The interns are tasked to design a training module on this topic to be conducted by the staff.
>
> Elizabeth and Stacy want to conduct a literature review so they can better understand the practice problem and learn from any similar experiences encountered by other researchers. They start with the following keywords: cooperation, biological parents, foster parents. But then what?
>
> In this case, the following questions can guide the process of finding appropriate literature:
>
> What are the specific times when biological and foster parents need to interact and for which they are most prepared?
>
> What do we exactly mean in this context by the terms "foster care," "cooperation," and "training"?
>
> How about other related topics? For example, what does the literature say about "loyalty," "role differentiation," "mutual acknowledgement," "attachment," and "roles and responsibilities" of biological and foster parents?

Conducting an Appropriate Literature Review

1. Sketch and illustrate the practice problem based on your knowledge and the results of the previous associative techniques.

2. Search for scientific articles and professional materials relevant to the practice problems by exploring various credible sources using key terms that represent the themes depicted in your sketch.

3. Review the materials and make summary notes of key points that describe important concepts, themes, and sub-themes as well as any interactions among them.

4. Summarize the key points on an evidence table or in a matrix.

An example matrix summarizing key information of a literature review related to a practice problem on smoking cessation interventions is given in table 2.3.

Technique 6: Stakeholder Identification

This technique helps you identify those players who are directly or indirectly involved in your practice problem.

Identifying Stakeholders

1. List different groups of stakeholders who could benefit from addressing the practice problem.

2. Describe each group of stakeholders and identify their roles in the practice problem

3. Summarize the results in a stakeholder identification matrix (table 2.4)

Technique 7: Changing the Perspective

Your experience of a practice problem differs from others' experiences of it. There are many people inside and outside of the organization who deal with your practice problem. This technique helps you identify and understand their views by analyzing the issue from different angles.

Exploring Other Perspectives

1. Briefly describe the way you see the practice problem, its causes, and why it needs to be addressed.

2. List people and/or groups inside and outside of your organization who are affected by the problem either directly (clients/patients, parents, caregivers, board members, etc.) or indirectly (journalists, politicians, community members, etc.).

3. Select a person or a group from the list and describe the practice problem from that point of view (i.e., perceptions of the cause, importance, and the solution). This may require you to contact people to find out more about their perspectives.

Themes and sub-themes	Sources and methods	Findings and notes
Smoking cessation, intervention, provider	Peer-delivered smoking counseling for childhood cancer survivors; Emmons et al. (2005). A randomized control trial with follow-up at 8 and 12 months that involved smokers (n = 796) enrolled onto the Childhood Cancer Survivors Study (CCSS) cohort.	This study suggests that the quit rate was significantly higher in the counseling group compared with the self-help group at both the 8-month (16.8% vs. 8.5%; P < .01) and 12-month follow-ups (15% vs. 9%; P < or = .01). This study also found that for 8-month follow-ups, there was a 5% increase in quit rate among those who received six calls compared with those who received five calls, 29% vs. 24% respectively.
Smoking cessation, intervention, behavior	Evaluating the effectiveness of a single telephone contact as an adjunct to a self-help intervention for smoking cessation; Míguez and Becoña (2008).	The study found that the point-prevalence abstinence rate was significantly higher in the telephone-support group than in the self-help-only group at the end of treatment (44.9% vs. 21.8%) and at the 3-month follow-up (39.0% vs. 26.4%).
Smoking cessation, intervention, behavior, target group	Smoking cessation, parents of young children; Abdullah et al. (2007). To evaluate the effectiveness of telephone counselling based on the stages of change.	The study found that the 7-day point prevalence abstinence rate at 6-month follow-up was significantly greater in the intervention group (15.3%; 68/444) than the control group (7.4%; 34/459) (P < 0.001).
Smoking cessation, intervention, behavior	Behavioral interventions as adjuncts to pharmacotherapy for smoking cessation; Stead and Lancaster (2012). To evaluate the effect of increasing the intensity of behavioral support for people who used medication for smoking cessation.	The study showed that increasing the amount of behavioral support was likely to increase the chance of success by about 10% to 25%, based on a pooled estimate from 38 trials. Subgroup analysis showed that there may be smaller benefit from providing even more intensive support for those who had at least 30 minutes of personal contact.
Smoking cessation, intervention, behavior, provider	Telephone counseling for smoking cessation: Effects of single-session and multiple-session interventions; Zhu et al. (1996). There were 3,030 study participants randomized into three groups.	Counseling groups had higher abstinence rates than self-help groups. The rates for having quit for at least 12 months by intention to treat were 5.4% for self-help, 7.5% for single counseling, and 9.9% for multiple counseling.
Smoking cessation practice guidelines, NASW	Implementing smoking cessation into your social work practice; Dorn (2017), National Association of Social Workers (NASW).	Identifies key principles for implementing cessation support as part of social work practice and identifies several evaluated programs for smoking cessation.
Smoking cessation practice guidelines, RNAO	Integrating tobacco interventions into daily practice; Registered Nurses' Association of Ontario (RNAO) (2017).	Practice recommendations: directed primarily to nurses and other health care providers in interprofessional teams who provide direct care to people in health system settings.
Smoking prevention and treatment guidelines, ENSP	ENSP guidelines for treating tobacco dependence; European Network for Smoking and Tobacco Prevention (ENSP) (2016).	Comprehensive guidelines for various forms of intervention in different settings.

Table 2.4. Example of a stakeholder identification matrix	
Stakeholders	Explanation
Social workers	A group of six supervisors (including myself) who support formerly homeless people. The social workers visit the clients at their homes and offer guidance with financial matters, substance abuse, employment, and functioning in a household.
Team leader	The team leader supervises the group and supports the clients.
Clients	These are adults who for various reasons were homeless and have been living independently for a while. They have applied and are eligible for receiving services. There are approximately 90 clients.

4. Repeat the previous step for other individuals and groups on your list.

5. Mark phrases and words with important information about the problem and look for potential connections and patterns among them.

Technique 8: Clarifying Assumptions

There are many ideas, thoughts, and assumptions around a practice problem, some of them controversial. Therefore, it is important to identify those assumptions. Here we define assumptions as personal interpretations of situations in the professional practice. Some assumptions can be in the form of common beliefs or stereotypes (e.g., a sedentary lifestyle can kill you the way that smoking does). Other assumptions might be in the form of clichés (e.g., if you work hard you can accomplish anything you want). Imagine that your practice problem is about biological parents who are concerned with the quality of services at a foster care center. You might make the following assumptions based on your past experiences and your knowledge of the literature:

- The staff and the parents want what is best for the child.
- The child benefits if the relationship between the parents and the center is good.
- The staff of the center are experienced and they know the right thing to do.
- The biological parents lost their rights to guardianship for a reason.

By charting your and other peoples' assumptions about the practice problem, you can better analyze and understand them.

Clarifying Different Assumptions

1. In a few sentences, briefly describe your own assumptions about the practice problem.

2. Invite the inside and outside stakeholders (e.g., parents, staff, board members, caregivers) to discuss the practice problem.

3. Explain the practice problem in objective and factual terms without sharing your own assumptions.

4. Give examples of assumptions that are not related to your practice problem (i.e., commonly accepted stereotypes and clichés) so the stakeholders understand what they need to do.

5. Give participants enough time so they can write down all their assumptions about the practice problem.

6. Mark words and phrases with important information and identify any connections or patterns either individually or in a group.

Technique 9: Collecting Data from the Place of Practice

This last technique is about gathering useful information in your professional practice by reviewing relevant documents, observing events, and/or interviewing key informants (i.e., stakeholders with useful knowledge and/or prior experience with the practice problem). Conducting research in your professional setting can provide you with ample opportunities for collecting data. To begin the process, you need to try to understand the main points related to your problem by reviewing internal documents such as organizational policies, protocols, logs, reports, meeting notes, and the like. If you have an observable practice problem (e.g., patient-provider interaction), you will gain firsthand insights about the problem by systematically observing relevant events.

Keep in mind, however, not all practice problems occur frequently enough to observe them and some are not readily seen. For example, problems such as poor communication, rare conflicts, and treatment challenges cannot be easily identified by an external observer. But you can gain valuable knowledge by interviewing those with relevant past experiences. Your interviews could be conducted formally (meetings, office interviews) or informally (lunch breaks, therapy sessions).

At this early stage of your practitioner research, these approaches are still exploratory and aimed at generating substantial amounts of descriptive information.

Reviewing and Analyzing Internal Documents and Data Sources

1. Briefly describe the practice problem in a few sentences.

2. Generate a list of topics related to the practice problem and prepare to extract relevant information in the form of questions or statements.

3. Index any available sources that you explore (clinical data, reports, etc.).

4. Look for the information that you need by reviewing the indexed sources.

5. Mark the important information and identify any connections and patterns among the phrases and concepts.

Performing an Observation

1. Briefly describe the practice problem in a few sentences.

2. Generate a list of specific occasions where the practice problem could be observed.

3. Sort the items on your list by their relevance and according to your availability and time commitment (e.g., how much time the observation requires vs. how much time you would be available).

4. Schedule the observation sessions that are most practical and valuable.

5. Perform your observation by trying to provide answers to the following questions: When exactly does the practice problem occur? How do different actors react to the problem? What are some of the specific circumstances of the event?

6. Write down your answers and mark phrases or words with important information; identify any connections or patterns.

Conducting Key Informant Interviews

1. Briefly describe the practice problem in a few sentences.

2. Generate a list of individuals and/or groups who are either directly or indirectly affected by your practice problem.

3. Identify those representatives whom you could meet and interview.

4. Plan your dates, times, and types of interviews (formal, informal).

5. Perform your interviews by trying to provide answers to the following questions: When exactly does the practice problem occur? How do different actors react to the problem? What are some of the specific circumstances of the event?

6. Prepare a detailed report and send it to the interviewees for approval and validation.

7. Mark phrases and words with important information individually or with your interviewee; identify any connections or patterns.

The three methods listed under technique 9 are discussed in more detail in chapters 3, 4, and 5.

Exercise 3. Exploring the Practice Problem (see page 62)

2.6. Describing the Practice Problem

After following the previously covered steps and techniques while exploring your problem idea, you will need to integrate all of the information into a revised and well-described practice problem. One systematic way to define your problem is through answering the following questions, known as the "6W+H method."

- What is the problem?
- Who is affected by the problem?
- When does the problem occur?
- Why is this a problem?
- Where does the problem occur?
- How did the problem begin?
- What is known about the solution of the problem?

You should be able to answer these questions using the information collected through your exploratory problem analysis. You may need to continue your exploration until you feel that you have enough information for answering the 6W+H questions.

While answering the questions, make sure that you properly and consistently cite your references according to a standard style (see appendix). It is also helpful to provide standard definitions of the key terms (e.g., patient participation, palliative care) and cite their sources, if applicable.

Answering the 6W+H Questions

First organize all the information that you have gathered in a way that is easily accessible, and then answer the questions based on your data to validate your understanding of the practice problem. Each question is followed by a few sub-questions. You may choose to use one or more of these sub-questions to answer your main question.

1. *What is the practice problem?*
   Provide a clear description.
   - Are there any specific irregularities or difficulties?
   - Are there any issues or situations deemed undesirable or unacceptable?
   - Are there any overlooked issues or components?
   - Are there any successful aspects of the practice that could or should be scaled up?

   You can use techniques such as mind mapping or concept mapping to answer the questions and clarify your practice problem.

2. *Who is affected by the problem?*
   Identify those individuals or groups that are affected by the practice problem.
   - Who are the people involved in the process? Who are the stakeholders?
   - What are their roles related to the practice problem?
   - What are the stakeholders' perceptions of the practice problem?

   You may want to include your stakeholder identification matrix here.

3. *When does the problem occur?*
   Indicate when and under which circumstances the practice problem occurs.
   - How frequently does the problem occur?
   - At what specific moments or circumstances does the problem occur?

4. *Why is this a problem?*
   Explain how the organization benefits from solving the problem.
   - Are there any quality standards or priorities that the organization is required to meet?
   - What types of benefits could be achieved by solving the problem?

5. *Where does the problem occur?*
   Identify the specific location(s) and circumstances surrounding the problem.

- In which physical area(s) does the problem occur?
- Under which circumstances does the problem occur?

6. *How did the problem begin?*
   - Explain the background and history of the problem.
   - What is the source of the problem?
   - What events preceded the problem?

   You may want to use a flowchart or a logic model to further clarify and visually demonstrate the answers.

7. *What is known about the solution of the problem?*
   - What has been done in the past to solve the problem and why haven't those efforts been sufficient?
   - What other solutions have stakeholders suggested?
   - Is it possible to control or solve the problem?
   - How have other organizations addressed similar problems? How much success have they had?

Defining the problem occasionally leads to some immediate actions, such as hiring a new staff member, better planning to avoid scheduling conflicts, or purchasing new equipment to improve safety. Going through the key components of practitioner research described in the next chapters will help you verify if and to what extent any of those actions worked.

Exercise 4. Developing a Concept Map and Conducting a Literature Review on a Hypothetical Practice Problem (see page 62)

Exercise 5. Literature Review (see page 62)

2.7. Documenting the Results

When you have finished the orientation step of the Practitioner Research Method, document your results according to the following list:

Motivation: Clearly describe the reason for conducting your research. Why and by whom have you been approached to carry out this project? Why did you decide to research this issue? Who will benefit from the results?

Context and relevance: Broadly define the context and setting of your research. Describe any specific characteristics of the organization and its environment that are relevant to your research. Explain to what extent your project is aligned with and relevant to the organization's mission, policies, and past research activities.

Literature review: Give a brief report of previous studies conducted on relevant concepts, themes, and sub-themes related to your practice problem and make sure that you correctly cite the sources of your information.

First version of the practice problem: Finalize the description of your practice problem using your answers to the 6W+H questions and their respective sub-questions.

Present the results to your stakeholders and other relevant parties in your organization to validate your findings and increase their engagement. Later you will learn how to integrate the results into parts A and B of your research plan.

2.8. Summary

Practitioner research can have multiple sources of motivation arising from different levels. You can clarify your motivation by explaining who encouraged you or requested your research and how the results benefit different stakeholders.

The term "practice problem" refers to all situations arising in professional practice that may become a starting point for in-depth studies and can be classified in the following categories: uncertainty, challenges, enhancement, learning, validation, anticipation, sustainability, and dissemination and scalability.

The practice problem is not always clearly defined when you start your research. There are several useful techniques that can help you identify a practice problem that interests you, such as brainstorming, keeping a journal, developing reflective reports, observation by others, and group discussions.

Once you identify a suitable topic, you can use exploratory analysis to develop a clearer understanding of the practice problem. Several techniques have been described that can help you systematically explore the practice problem, such as brainstorming about the practice problem, mind mapping, concept mapping, journaling, changing the perspective, identifying stakeholders, and clarifying assumptions. Reviewing the literature and collecting data in your professional practice can supplement these techniques.

The 6W+H questions can guide you through the process of using your collected information to define the practice problem. Those questions are:

- What is the problem?
- Who is affected by the problem?
- When does the problem occur?
- Why is this a problem?
- Where does the problem occur?
- How did the problem begin?
- What is known about the solution of the problem?

Lastly, document and organize your findings and present them to your stakeholders and other relevant parties in your organization. Later, when it's time to write your research plan, you will learn how to use the definition of the practice problem to inform the process.

Exercise 1. Identifying Suitable Practice Problems

Six techniques are described on pages 43–46 that can help you identify potential practice problems in your professional setting. Practice at least one technique and discuss the findings with your other team members (e.g., colleagues, client/patients, fellow students, etc.).

Exercise 2. Create Your Own Set of Criteria

Create your own set of criteria for identifying and prioritizing practice problems. Discuss this list with important stakeholders.

Exercise 3. Exploring the Practice Problem

Nine techniques are described on pages 49–58 to help you explore and analyze the practice problem. Practice at least one technique and discuss the findings with your other team members (e.g., colleagues, clients/patients, fellow students, etc.).

Exercise 4. Developing a Concept Map and Conducting a Literature Review on a Hypothetical Practice Problem

The purpose of this exercise is to help you better understand how concept mapping guided by published literature can enhance your understanding of a practice problem. As a group, choose a hypothetical practice problem that you are all interested in exploring. Either individually or collectively, create a concept map that captures your assumptions about the causes of the problem. Next, everyone commits to finding suitable information on the topics in the concept map. When you complete your individual assignments, meet as a group and share what you have learned. Finish the discussion by reflecting on the new insights that you have gained about the practice problem.

Exercise 5. Literature Review

An organization plans to design a self-management training program for a specific group of patients. Choose a group of patients with specific characteristics (e.g., type II diabetes) as a target population. Each member of your team will be tasked to find and review at least three scientific sources on different aspects of self-management relevant to your target patients. Ascertain to what extent your previous assumptions about this subject are either confirmed or invalidated by the literature. Discuss and reflect on your findings in the group.

REFERENCES

Abdullah, A. S. M., Mak, Y. W., Loke, A. Y., & Lam, T. H. (2005). Smoking cessation intervention in parents of young children: A randomised controlled trial. *Addiction*, *100*(11), 1731–1740.

Buzan, T. (2003). *The Mind Map Book*. BBC Books.

Dorn, C. (2017). *Practice perspectives: Implementing smoking cessation into your social work practice*. National Association of Social Workers. https://www.socialworkers.org/LinkClick.aspx?fileticket=aBwsL4z4nC0%3D&portalid=0

Emmons, K. M., et al. (2005). Peer-delivered smoking counseling for childhood cancer survivors increases rate of cessation: The partnership for health study. *Journal of Clinical Oncology*, *23*(27), 6516–6523.

European Network for Smoking and Tobacco Prevention. (2016). *ENSP guidelines for treating tobacco dependence*. https://www.europeanpublishing.eu/2016ebooks

Geenen, M. (2017). *Reflecteren. Leren van je ervaringen als sociale professional* [Reflection: Learning from your experiences as a social work professional]. Coutinho.

Míguez, M. C., & Becoña, E. (2008). Evaluating the effectiveness of a single telephone contact as an adjunct to a self-help intervention for smoking cessation in a randomized controlled trial. *Nicotine & Tobacco Research*, *10*(1), 129–135.

Registered Nurses' Association of Ontario. (2017). *Integrating tobacco interventions into daily practice*. (3rd ed.). https://rnao.ca/sites/rnao-ca/files/bpg/RNAO_Integrating_Tobacco_Interventions_into_Daily_Practice_2017_Third_Edition_Best_Practice_Guideline_0.pdf

Stead, L. F., & Lancaster, T. (2012). Behavioural interventions as adjuncts to pharmacotherapy for smoking cessation. *Cochrane Database of Systematic Reviews*, (12), CD009670.

Zhu, S. H., Stretch, V., Balabanis, M., Rosbrook, B., Sadler, G., & Pierce, J. P. (1996). Telephone counseling for smoking cessation: Effects of single-session and multiple-session interventions. *Journal of Consulting and Clinical Psychology*, *64*(1), 202.

3

Focusing

Focusing is the key component of the Practitioner Research Method that helps you delve into more in-depth problem analysis based on theoretical frameworks and empirical data (figure 3.1). In this stage, you will expand your knowledge about the scientific and professional literature on your identified practice problem.

This chapter will systematically guide you through effective focusing by first teaching you how to perform an in-depth problem analysis. The results of your problem analysis will provide the information you need to formulate your research objectives. Your objectives help you clarify realistic expectations for what you intend to achieve. In addition, they can guide you through understanding what is known and asking questions that are not yet answered.

Formulating your main research question is the next step in the focusing process. Having a well-articulated research question determines the scope of the research and enables you to be more systematic in planning your activities. You will go through the process of identifying important sub-questions and evaluating their validity.

At the end of this chapter, we provide a brief summary of concepts and relevant exercises.

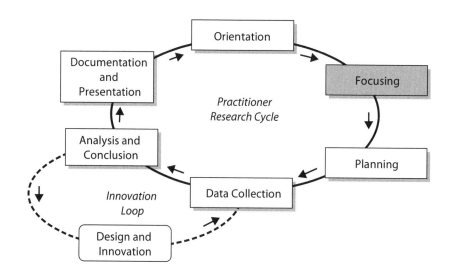

Figure 3.1

Key component of practitioner research: Focusing

3.1. In-Depth Problem Analysis

During the orientation stage, you examined the practice problem from various angles. For the focusing stage, the overall intention is to further explore your practice problem using the scientific and professional literature and to come up with a *conceptual framework* for your research. A good literature review entails certain features that lead to using those scientific findings to better formulate and communicate your research questions.

What is a Literature Review?

A literature review is an organized effort to identify and study published scientific and professional information for the purpose of learning from the results of previous inquiries in the areas related to your practice problem. A good literature review will help you define and outline key concepts of your practitioner research study. In addition, learning from previous studies will help you identify the underlying theories that could shape your study's conceptual framework. A successful literature review will help you define and fine-tune your research objectives and questions.

In professional practice, every problem is somehow unique and bound to specific contextual characteristics. Therefore, a good literature review has two main characteristics. First, the information and sources that you review should be relevant to the specific nature and context of your practice problem. You and your colleagues, as practitioner researchers, have autonomy over defining what is relevant. Second, the literature you cite should come from sources that are trustworthy, which is often defined by criteria such as being peer-reviewed, published in high-impact journals, and/or endorsed by credible and widely respected organizations or individuals. Further, it is good practice to include literature from more than one disciplinary perspective (e.g., psychology, sociology, biology) relevant to your research.

A literature review can inform the other stages of the Practitioner Research Method in the following ways:

- You can use what you learn from reviewing the literature to inform your data collection methods (chapter 4). You may learn how to construct the tools and instruments you'll need, such as comparison charts, observation and response charts, interview guides, questionnaires, and the like.

- A thorough review of the literature can significantly save you time and resources during data collection as well if you are able to identify existing research findings that address your research issue.

- Your literature review findings can guide your analysis and conclusions (chapter 6) by helping you better understand and categorize your data and draw compelling insights from your research.

- For design research (chapter 7), any information found about similar interventions may support you in making informed decisions about your research process. In addition, you can make use of literature to validate the principles on which your design is based.

How to Conduct a Literature Review

The literature review starts with your exploratory problem analysis, as discussed in section 2.5 (technique 5: review of the literature). A good literature review is a continuous effort that helps to focus your practice problem and to document and implement your findings. Information gained through this process is useful for describing the practice problem, based on professional and scientific evidence using the 6W+H method (see section 2.6). Here you will learn the step-by-step process for using scientific and professional sources to increase your academic and practical knowledge about your practice problem. The features of a good literature review for practitioner research—including types of print and online sources, strategies for finding the needed sources, how to assess the credibility of your identified sources, and referencing formats—is outlined in the appendix.

To start, your literature review should aim to focus on the following five domains of your practice problem: (1) definition, (2) consequences, (3) frequency and severity, (4) possible causes and history, and (5) solutions and improvement strategies. Focusing on these domains of your practice problem will help you stay highly selective of sources with the greatest potential to add value to your research, and the results of your literature review will in turn help you refine your practice problem.

There are several questions based on these practice problem domains that can help you identify the most appropriate literature for your research. This is not an exhaustive set of questions, so feel free to include additional relevant questions under each domain or disregard questions that are not relevant to your particular practice problem:

Definition of the Practice Problem

How is the practice problem described or defined in the literature or in professional practice?

What are the main components and sub-components of the practice problem?

What are the key theoretical concepts, themes, and sub-themes used to describe the problem?

How do different components and sub-components of the problem interact?

How is a practice problem most often recognized and identified?

What are the characteristics and criteria used to identify the problem?

What are some of the specific examples and cases used to describe and define the problem?

What are the similarities and differences between different descriptions of the problem in the literature?

Consequences of the Practice Problem

Which individuals and groups are affected by the practice problem (e.g., clients/patients, colleagues, administrators)? How are they affected? In what situations?

How do people in different situations perceive and react to the problem?

What are the major concerns of each individual and group?

How are their concerns and reactions related to their role or background?

In which specific situations is the practice problem noticeable and why?

What are the short-, mid-, and long-term effects of the problem?

What is the impact of the problem on professional and clinical practice?

What is the impact of the problem at the organizational level?

What is the impact of the problem at the community and policy levels?

Frequency and Severity of the Practice Problem

What are the specific moments that the practice problem occurs?

How frequently does the practice problem occur?

What are stages and levels of severity when the problem occurs?

How critical can the situation get?

What are some of the worst possible consequences and ramifications of the problem?

Possible Causes and History of the Practice Problem

Why does the problem occur? What are some of the possible causes or factors associated with the occurrence of the problem?

What circumstances influence the emergence of the practice problem?

What circumstances precede the practice problem?

What reasons are put forward as the cause of the emergence of the practice problem?

How does the problem usually develop over time if not resolved?

Solutions and Improvement Strategies for the Practice Problem

What solutions to the practice problem does the literature provide?

How can the practice problem be prevented?

What are the strategies to alleviate and moderate the practice problem?

What are some of the key characteristics of improvement strategies and their areas of impact?

What is the level of scientific evidence for the effectiveness of these improvement strategies?

After finding relevant sources, the next step is to review them and summarize key points. Some techniques commonly used for organizing these summaries include (1) creating a summary of important notes for each source, (2) organizing the notes in a matrix along with some reference information (e.g., author names, publication date), (3) annotating the paper-based or electronic files of the sources, and (4) classifying the information in an outline format according to its relevance to your practitioner research study. Reference information can be organized through specialized software (e.g., Reference Manager, EndNote, Zotero) or in spreadsheets. Using citation management software can make it a lot easier for you to use relevant sources in publications and simplifies changing the citation format when needed.

The last step in a literature review is synthesizing your summary notes. Develop an outline using your main topics and order them according to the logical flow of your argument (e.g., introduction, statement of the practice problem, comparing theories and pro-

Table 3.1. Outline for a literature review		
Topic	Purpose	Detailed content
Introduction	Explain the rationale and justification for conducting the literature review	Significance of the practice problem; gaps in the literature; objective of the literature review

Practice problem	Describe the practice problem according to the published literature	Significance, description, and scope
		    How is the practice problem described or defined?
		    Which groups or individuals have commonly suffered from the practice problem?
		    When and how does the practice problem occur?
		Consequences and progression
		    What are some of the consequences of the practice problem?
		    What are some common ways the practice problem emerges?
		Solutions
		    What are some of the solutions or improvement strategies offered to address the practice problem?

Differences and similarities	Compare sources to identify agreement or disagreement between their findings	What are some of the differences and similarities in the results and conclusions provided by the sources? How can I use this information to better inform the practitioner research study? How can I deal with contradictory results and perspectives?
Comparison between theories and professional practice	Compare original description of the practice problem based on personal experience with descriptions of the practice problem according to the literature	What are some of the differences between my description of the practice problem and that in the literature? How does the literature relate to how the stakeholders view the practice problem? Which aspects of the practice problem have not yet been fully addressed in the literature? What are some of the limitations of my literature review?
Discussions and conclusion	Discuss the findings and draw conclusions on how best to plan the practitioner research study	What are some of the logical assumptions that can be made based on the results? What would be the main conclusions? Which conclusion will add more value to my project, and why? What are the implications of the discussion and conclusion of my practitioner research study?

fessional practice, discussion, and conclusion). An outline helps you see the big picture and then identify important subheadings and details. For further exploration of the topics, describe the purpose of each topic (i.e., how do they contribute to your literature review?) and list details and guiding questions under each topic in an orderly fashion.

Sometimes, as part of the process, you find sources with contradictory findings and arguments. In such cases, you often need to decide—based on your own and your stakeholders' judgments—which findings are more useful and relevant to your project. Lastly, it often occurs that a more in-depth literature review results in new findings that lead you to change the way you characterize the initial practice problem. That's why following the Practitioner Research Method usually requires going back to previous stages, revising the practice problem, and revisiting the orientation stage. An example of what to include in an outline in order to synthesize the information gained through a literature review is provided in table 3.1.

Exercise 1. Searching the Literature: Finding Useful Textual Sources (see page 90)

Exercise 2. Prepare for the Literature Review: Link the Concepts with Sources (see page 90)

3.2. Formulating Research Objectives

As discussed earlier, the goal of practitioner research is to offer a solution to a practice problem and improve the quality and effectiveness of health care and social services. A clear research objective is an indication of what exactly you want to achieve with your findings. Your objectives specify what you want to add to current knowledge and insights pertaining to the practice problem as well as the practical solutions to the problem you would like to develop by translating your findings into feasible applications. The findings of practitioner research can be varied and diverse in nature, covering such topics as defining standards of care for the provided services, streamlining individualized care, improving diagnostic practices, creating healing and welcoming practice environments, and providing evidence for intervention effects under unique conditions. The more you narrow down your objectives, the simpler and more practical it becomes to come up with effective solutions. In addition, more focused objectives can help you better communicate your research to your colleagues and open the door to constructive dialogue and teamwork. You may choose research objectives that are near and dear to your heart, but keep in mind the objectives should add value to professional practice, either directly or indirectly, so you can be supported and succeed. The difference between the direct and indirect relevance of your research objectives to professional practice are illustrated in the following examples.

Example 1. A child psychiatrist is very interested in learning what impact her treatments have on the emotional well-being of her patients at the time of their termination. She plans a practitioner research study to learn about her patients' experiences by first conducting individual in-depth interviews with three patients as a pilot assessment. The primary objective for conducting this study is personal; she wants to know how well she has been able to meet the needs of her patients.

This objective can indirectly affect her colleagues as many of them might be interested in gaining similar knowledge. But, more importantly, the research objective is directly aligned with the overall organization's agenda of improving the quality and effectiveness of treatment services. In this case, our practitioner researcher is in a win-win situation as her research objective is aligned with both her personal and organizational interests.

Example 2. The supervising nurse of a child psychiatry department is directed by the management team to use practitioner research to assess and evaluate the patient discharge process, with the objective of improving the process. At first, our practitioner researcher is not personally engaged in the assignment. However, after conducting a thorough literature review, she realizes that improving the discharge process could reveal critical information about the effectiveness of health care services that, if shared with the health care staff, could lead to significant quality improvement, an objective that does engage her.

Well-defined objectives also determine the direction of your practitioner research and contribute to the formulation of informative research questions.

Example. A nonprofit organization has started a youth after-school program for inner-city girls in grades 6–8 that includes life skills and social and emotional development activities. The program has been very well received by the local community. A public health intern working with the organization intends to conduct a practitioner research study with the objective of learning effective ways to increase the number of participants by up to 20 percent in six months. Several related research questions could be formulated: How much do parents, schools, and kids know about the program? What are the factors that could influence the youths' decisions to join the program? What roles can parents play in motivating their kids to join the program? How well does the organization involve their current participants, their parents, and other partners in advertising and promoting the program?

Answers to each of these questions helps achieve the research objective. However, answering research questions requires a commitment of time and resources. Your literature review and other activities related to focusing your practice problem could inform your decisions about what specific areas your research would cover and why. For instance, the public health intern in our last example might find certain questions relevant to the research objective but not quite aligned with the kind of focus and boundaries that he wants to set for his project:

How can we include the policy makers and leaders of other organizations in promoting the youth program?

How can we raise funds to modernize the youth center and improve the quality of the program?

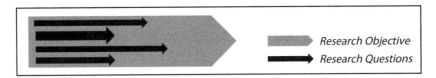

Research Objective
Research Questions

Figure 3.2

Research questions must fall within the scope of the research objective

A responsive research question must be aligned with the stated research objective *and* within the scope of your project (see figure 3.2). Therefore, having relevant and well-formulated research questions is a major step in helping you focus on what's needed for your practitioner research study.

The following five guidelines can help you formulate and fine-tune your research objectives.

Guideline 1: Defining the Research Objective Following a Problem Analysis

Analyzing your practice problem is the most practical and appropriate way to learn what exactly you need to know and achieve in your practitioner research study. You need to analyze the practice problem from practical and theoretical perspectives in terms of the areas that are known as well as the gaps in understanding. A good research objective is a balanced statement addressing both scientific and professional knowledge you intend to gain with the ultimate purpose of addressing the practice problem. Here your job is to clarify what aspects of the practice problem you want to focus on and investigate by formulating a descriptive and specific research objective.

Guideline 2: Describing the Research Objective as an Outcome

Your research objective is indicative of the kind of knowledge you want to gain after implementing the study. Here there are two types of expected outcomes that you need to be able to differentiate:

1. To gain new insights and knowledge—sometimes requested by an agency or institution—to better understand the situation and fill a knowledge gap.
2. To improve the quality and effectiveness of the professional practice by improving current interventions or designing and testing a new one.

Guideline 3: Stating the Research Objective as Clearly and Unambiguously as Possible

In the following example, a research objective is vaguely defined:

A community hospital would like to improve their visitation policy in a reasonable time frame.

In a statement like this, readers can come up with various interpretations, making it hard to generate focused research questions. The terms "in a reasonable time frame" and "improve" are relative, subjective, and not quite clear; they are open to personal interpretations, and it would be difficult for your colleagues to clearly understand what you mean by them. Consequently, this makes it harder for your colleagues to give you useful feedback on your research plan. Other terms, such as "eventually," "good," and "quickly," have the same problem of ambiguity and it's best to avoid those as well. A more useful and concrete formulation would be:

> Over the next six months, the community hospital administrators and staff will review and revise the guidelines set forth in the visitation policy to minimize interruption of clinical services.

In this revised statement, the objective specifies the task of working on a specific policy. It is always a good idea to explain terms that might get interpreted in different ways by different people. This can apply to the terms "visitation policy," "guidelines," and "interruption" here.

Guideline 4: Demonstrating the Relevance of the Research Objective to Practitioner Research

A practitioner research objective should be achievable within its organizational context and have the potential to improve the professional practice. Therefore, it should include relevant phrases about the context and contributions of the research objective to the professional practice, which is different than objectives for research that has a more academic focus.

Guideline 5: Revising the Research Objective Based on Input from the Stakeholders

You can significantly strengthen and improve the clarity of your research objective by sharing it with your colleagues and soliciting their feedback; you can discuss every assumption and generate consensus around the wording of your research objective. Other stakeholders often have ideas and assumptions about your research and its expected results that are different than yours. A good research objective is one that gives each stakeholder a similar understanding of your proposed research goals.

Exercise 3. Research Objectives (see page 90)

3.3. Identifying Research Questions

Research questions and research objectives form the foundation of your practitioner research study, so it is critical that they both are stated as clearly and unambiguously as possible. However, there is no straightforward pathway to identify questions that are succinct, specific, and relevant to what you are trying to discover through your research. The process requires identifying questions, reflecting on them, and making revisions.

You can save yourself lots of frustration if you invest the needed time for identifying good research questions and pay attention to the details that could improve the relevance and clarity of your questions. Having good research questions will ultimately make it easier for you to plan your study, collect data, and analyze your findings.

Here are five techniques that can help you identify appropriate research questions. You can use the techniques individually or as a group. However, doing this in a diverse group of stakeholders would help you generate more ideas and enhance the level of support for your research. Here the main goal is to identify a large number of relevant questions that could be later reviewed and reduced to those that are most appropriate and feasible.

Technique 1: Use Question (Interrogative) Words

Use appropriate question words to examine various inquiries relevant to your research objective:

1. Review the results of your problem analysis and your stated research objective.

2. List question (interrogative) words "who," "what," "when," "where," "which," "why," "how," and "to what extent."

3. Draft questions using your question words while thinking about your research objective and problem analysis. At this point, don't be concerned about the validity of the questions; you will review them later.

Technique 2: Brainstorm

Practice problems are usually multifaceted and have various components and sub-components that could inform and inspire research questions. As a researcher, you are in charge of deciding what questions to focus on and which ones to leave unexplored.

1. Review your problem analysis and research objective to refresh your memory.

2. Highlight various components and sub-components of the practice problem that are aligned with your research objective and that emerged from the problem analysis.

3. Try to brainstorm either individually or in a group to generate as many questions as possible on two or three selected components or sub-components of your practice problem.

4. Repeat this process for other components or sub-components, if needed.

Technique 3. Compare Theory and Practice

One major concern in identifying practitioner research questions is about the relevance of the information gathered through your literature review to your professional context. If the information is not deemed relevant, then either it would be hard to use it to inform relevant research questions, or the relevance of the resulting questions might be questionable. This technique helps you address this potential problem from the start.

1. Review your problem analysis and research objective to refresh your memory
2. Write down every significant finding from the literature review that you think has questionable relevance to professional practice.
3. Try to examine the subject in ways that could illuminate potential links between the findings and professional practice.

Technique 4: Formulate Different Types of Research Questions

1. Review your problem analysis and research objective to refresh your memory.
2. Draw a table with five rows. Each row represents one type of question: descriptive, defining, comparative, evaluative, and explanatory.
3. Formulate a few questions for each question type based on your problem analysis and research objective. At this point, don't be concerned about the validity of the question; you will revisit that aspect later.

The various types of practitioner research questions and study designs—descriptive, defining, comparative, evaluative, and explanatory—were mentioned in chapter 1. As discussed, these categories are not mutually exclusive (e.g., an evaluation or design question can also be a descriptive question). Here, however, you can find examples of simple research questions under each of the aforementioned categories:

Descriptive questions (regarding the current status)

- What are the sociodemographic characteristics and health conditions of a community health center's patients?
- What are some of the most commonly reported issues around safety and security among practitioners at a rehabilitation center?
- What is the level of knowledge and experience among the staff of a nursing home about the specific needs of elderly suffering from a mental health condition?
- What is the flow of administrative activities and nursing services, from intake to discharge, provided to patients undergoing surgical operations in a city hospital?
- What is the frequency of using recommended evidence-based motivation enhancement techniques for smoking cessation among family physicians in a health care organization?
- What is the prevalence of past drug and alcohol use among students attending a community college, stratified by their sociodemographic characteristics and academic performance?

Descriptive questions (regarding possible improvements)

- What should a responsive education-training program for teenage pregnant girls look like?

- What would be the best approach for an ophthalmology clinic trying to provide culturally sensitive health care services for children of undocumented immigrants?
- How can indoor play materials be made more challenging for the participating autistic children in the health care center?
- What would be the best use of available technology to improve the intake process of a social service program?

Defining questions

- What is the interpretation of healthy living conditions among senior citizens suffering from cardiovascular diseases?
- How is the concept of children's engagement in sports operationalized in three Chicago inner-city neighborhoods?
- What does success of drug rehabilitation services provided at clients' homes mean from the informal caregivers' perspective?
- How do teenage mothers from various ethnic backgrounds define "independent living"?
- What do practitioners in our organization mean when they refer to "patient self-management"?

Comparative questions

- What are the comparative benefits and disadvantages of dental services being provided in renovated facilities versus nonrenovated facilities?
- What is the differential impact of an improvised music therapy program on patients diagnosed major depressive compared to those with anxiety disorders?
- What is the impact of intake interviews being conducted by a two-person team on clients' perceived quality of services and level of satisfaction compared to the standard of care?
- What effect does providing informational materials to patients diagnosed with type 2 diabetes have on their reported self-care behaviors compared to those who only receive standard services?

Evaluative questions

- What is the level of compliance with the new visitation policy among foster care counselors, guardians, children, and biological parents?
- What do school teachers and administrators think about the local community's after-school life skills training programs?
- How well is the HIV/AIDS prevention curriculum implemented by the personnel of the HIV testing and counseling mobile units?
- What is the impact of the new aftercare protocol for treating youth with alcohol intoxication on their attitudes about binge drinking?
- How do teenagers aged 13 to 16 years old with physical disabilities rate the range of activities offered by the local YMCA recreation center?

- What are the best ways of using local homeless shelters' physical spaces for conducting needs assessment and training?

Explanatory questions

- Why did setting up strict rules for a particular group of youth lead to a decline in conflicts between the members?
- Why did several social services clients report not having strong confidence in their case manager?
- Why do male patients use the online services less frequently than female patients?
- Why did several nurses and doctors in emergency care not completely follow the recommended protective regulations?

Technique 5: Question Hierarchy

Questions are often ordered within a hierarchy. To answer a specific question, you often need to answer the question that logically precedes it. In addition, in answering a question you often generate further questions. This technique helps you evoke new questions and examine the question hierarchy in an engaging and simple manner.

1. Take a look at your problem analysis and your research objective.
2. Randomly pick a question related to your problem analysis and objective.
3. Write down questions that might be asked prior to this question, and also questions that could follow this question.
4. Generate new questions and repeat this process.

For example:

Questions prior to this question	Main Question	Questions that could follow this question
How are "the elderly" defined?	What are some of the differences between perceived loneliness among the elderly and teenagers?	How do these differences emerge?
What is "perceived loneliness"?		In what way could lonely elderly and lonely young people help each other?
How does loneliness manifest itself among the elderly and teenagers?		

Choosing the Most Appropriate Research Questions

At this point, you have compiled a list of possible research questions. Now it is time to select the questions that are most appropriate and could be answered by your practitioner research study. Examine each question from your list for the following criteria:

Is this question a logical result of the problem analysis?

Is this question aligned with the research objective?

Has this question been answered in previous studies in this particular context?

Do I have a personal interest in answering this question through practitioner research?

Are other stakeholders in my organization interested in this question?

What are my expected results from researching this question? Are they realistic?

Can this question be fully answered by conducting this practitioner research study?

Can this question be answered within the project's time limit and with available resources?

Exercise 4. Main Research Questions (see page 91)

3.4. Determining the Scope of the Research Question

The data needed to answer questions can vary significantly, as can the complexity of the methods for acquiring the data. As a result, some questions can be answered more quickly and easily than others with fewer resources. Hence, the guiding principle in analyzing the scope of your research question is whether or not a question can be answered in a given time frame and with a set amount of resources.

> *Example.* "What are the differences between male and female social work professionals?"

This question is broad and open to interpretation, making it impossible to collect and analyze data about every possible scenario in a reasonable time frame. Therefore, you will need to limit the scope of the question by stating it more specifically. For instance, the revised question can become something like this:

> "What are the differences between male and female social work professionals in the way they interview homeless clients?"

The question can be narrowed down even further:

> "What are the differences between male and female social work professionals in the way they interview homeless clients aged 60 and over?"

On the other hand, be careful not to state the question in a too highly specified manner. "How many homeless shelters are located in our inner-city neighborhood?" could be easily answered with an online search and does not qualify as a research question. The question could, however, be further broadened, such as "To what extent do homeless shelters in our inner-city neighborhood incorporate religious and ideological philosophies into their services and programs?" By broadening or tightening your questions, you can set the scope of your research question to focus on what you need and want to achieve. Two techniques here can help you set the scope of your research questions.

Technique 1: Zoom In and Out

Similar to viewing a Google map from your tablet, zooming out can help you view the big picture and zooming in provides you with more details. A similar concept can be used to determine the scope and level of detail covered by a practitioner research question. The limits of the research question can be explored by broadening it or tightening it, and the process can be informed by using information acquired through your problem analysis and literature review.

1. Write down the latest version of your research question.
2. Focus on different aspects of your research question, such as:

    Actor(s): Who are the major players (e.g., internal and external stakeholders) in finding the answer to the research question?

    Target group: Which individuals or groups are the intended beneficiaries of the research and addressing the practice problem?

    Benefits: What knowledge, skills, or insights do you hope to gain by answering the question?

    Context: What specific professional practice settings does your research focus on?

    Professional services: What aspects of professional services are central to your research?

    Design research: What type of interventions do you intend to invent for improving the professional practice?

3. Zoom out (broaden your research question) by adding more general concepts to the current research question.
4. Zoom in (narrow down your research question) by writing more specific concepts than the one(s) covered in your research question.

By creating a table with these components (table 3.2), you and your colleagues can decide on the scope of the research question and formulate a question that is best suited to help you achieve the research objective in a given time frame with available resources.

Use the next technique to verify whether or not your question can be feasibly researched.

Technique 2: Thinking Forward

This technique helps you visualize the steps and the process required for your research in order to verify whether the research question is feasible and realistic.

1. Write down the latest version of your research question.
2. List all the specific results that your practitioner research may generate.
3. Think about the results and work your way down the list, mentally imagining the steps needed to reach each individual result.
4. Consider whether the necessary steps can be completed in the time frame allocated for the research. If not, you will need to make compromises by narrowing down your research question (zooming in).

Table 3.2 Zooming out and in on the original research question: "What is the quality of the HIV/AIDS prevention curriculum implemented by the personnel of the HIV testing and counseling mobile units?"

	Zoom out Level 2: Add . . .	Zoom out Level 1: Add . . .	Original Scope	Zoom in Level 1: Limit to . . .	Zoom in Level 2: Limit to . . .
Actors	Supervisors	Community workers	Staff at the mobile unit	Five students	Two students
Target group	Friends	Members of their households	People living with HIV/AIDS	People 18–30 years old	Males 18–30 years old
Benefits	More communication; less stigma	Less high-risk sexual behaviors; more supportive household	More knowledge gained; intention to engage in safe sexual practices	More knowledge on routes of HIV transmission	Awareness about safe sex practices
Context	Other local programs	Nearby community	Mobile HIV testing and counseling unit	Only testing and counseling activities	Only counseling
Services	Communication and marketing campaign	Community education	Health education and counseling	Only counseling	Only education
Design	Radio spots and social media messages	Informational materials	A checklist for assessing the quality of implementation	A counseling assessment checklist	An education assessment checklist

This technique is more useful if conducted in a group or at least in collaboration with another colleague. Ask others to give you feedback on your envisioned steps for achieving each intended result. This can help you be more accurate in your estimation of the scope of the research question.

Exercise 5. Determine the Scope of a Research Question (see page 91)

3.5. Subdividing the Research Question

Practitioner research mostly takes place in uncontrolled practice settings where research questions entail several components, some too complex and hard to be investigated in their entirety. Such questions often have layers of sub-questions that have to be answered before the primary questions can be answered. One solution is to divide the question into more straightforward, manageable sub-questions, each focused on easy-to-understand components of the main question. Each sub-question is like a piece of a jigsaw puzzle, which, when combined, could result in the answer to the overarching research question. Lastly, during data collection, you may come up with new sub-questions that you want to consider, which leads to revisiting the main research question and already identified sub-questions. This process illustrates the iterative nature of practitioner research.

Here we provide you with two examples to better understand the concept of sub-dividing the research question.

Main Question Example 1. How effective and relevant are job training services offered to low-income residents of Baltimore City by the Department of Social Services?

Sub-Questions

What professional development services does the department offer to the employees responsible for conducting the education and training?

What are the specific training needs of clients in the areas of GED (general education development) preparation, computer literacy, English for speakers of other languages (ESOL), résumé writing, job search, and interviewing skills?

How are the department's job training services mapped with the training needs of the clients?

What are the department's hallmarks of success? How are they measured and tracked?

Main Question Example 2. What are the potential areas for interdisciplinary collaboration between health care professionals affiliated with the Chicago Department of Public Health?

Sub-Questions

What are the potential areas for interdisciplinary collaboration in public health according to the literature?

What are some good examples of interdisciplinary collaboration in other health departments in the United States?

What is the current level and what are examples of interdisciplinary collaboration between the health care professionals in the department?

What are the intended results and outcomes of high-impact interdisciplinary collaborations among the health care professionals working at different levels of care?

The key principle is to verify that the combined answers to the sub-questions constitute a complete answer to the main question. If you think this may not be the case, you need to further explore the main question for any missing sub-questions. The same techniques that were introduced in sections 3.3 and 3.4 can be used for drafting and choosing the sub-questions. In addition, you can use the following techniques that are specifically relevant to the sub-questions.

Technique 1: Focused Brainstorming

This technique is very similar to "Technique 2: Brainstorm" from section 3.3. In this case, you only focus on relevant components of the main question and generate sub-questions associated with each component or with their interaction. This will help you gain further insights into the important unknown aspects of the main question.

1. Write down the main research question and the identified components and sub-components that emerged from the problem analysis and the research objective.

2. List those components associated with the key unknown areas related to your main question informed by the gaps identified in your literature review and the problem analysis.

3. Draft focused sub-questions relevant to each component with a more limited scope than the main question.

Example. A nurse practitioner working in a hospital is interested in conducting practitioner research with the following main question: "What is the impact of our counseling program on the quality of life of patients after open heart surgery?"

According to her literature review, "quality of life" comprises physical health, mental health, and social well-being. Therefore, to begin with, the following sub-questions can be stated for those components:

What is the impact of the counseling program on the patients' physical health?

What is the impact of the counseling program on the patients' mental health?

What is the impact of the counseling program on the patients' social well-being?

Technique 2: Stating the Sub-Questions from Different Perspectives

This technique helps you describe the sub-questions with different perspectives in mind, so the main question is answered according to the desires and the worldview of the target groups and stakeholders. This could include the perspectives of clients/patients, colleagues, physicians, nurses, social workers, or members of the community. Here you need to focus on the perspectives that are most relevant to the practice problem.

1. Write down the main research question.

2. List various perspectives relevant to the main question that you wish to explore.

3. Draft focused sub-questions from different perspectives with a more limited scope than the main question.

You may want to do this from all of the perspectives on your list for each of the sub-questions. Doing this technique with a diverse group of colleagues, partners, or clients/patients could further improve its effectiveness. In that case, you may draft the sub-questions and have your colleagues reflect on them or let everyone draft a few questions from different perspectives and then compare the results.

In the last example, the nurse practitioner wanted to assess the impact of the counseling program on patients' quality of life by including other perspectives, such as the patients, their partners, the health care team, and the community health workers. In this case, she can create a list of sub-questions, such as:

- What are the key aspects of quality of life from the patients' perspective? What do patients think is the impact of the counseling program on their quality of life?

- What are the key aspects of quality of life from the perspective of the patients' partners? What impact do their partners think the counseling program has on the quality of life of patients?

- What are the key aspects of quality of life from the perspective of the health care team? What impact does the health care team think the counseling program has on the quality of life of patients?

- What are the key aspects of quality of life from the perspective of community health workers? What impact do community health workers think the counseling program has on the quality of life of patients?

Different Levels of Sub-Questions

Sub-questions are not often at the same level and you would need to answer those that are more introductory before being able to answer the more advanced and specific ones; in other words, you cannot answer the next question before answering its prerequisites.

Example 1. You want to conduct a practitioner research study to design an orientation and training program responsive to the needs of your organization's new employees. Your main question is: What are the main differences between the newly hired counselors compared to their senior peers with at least 10 years of experience with regard to their level of knowledge about the organization and their professional competencies in counseling? The initial sub-question that you *need* to answer is: What are the basic insights and fundamental proficiencies needed for a counselor in your organization in order to succeed?

After answering that first sub-question, you can start working on finding the answers to other sub-questions, such as: What are some of the common misunderstandings and mistakes that new hires would make in their first few months on the job? What are some of the skills and techniques used by senior counselors to avoid mistakes such as those made by their junior peers?

Example 2. You're doing design research to answer the question "What would be the best intervention to motivate my colleagues to more actively engage in addressing the needs of patients suffering from dementia?" You start by contemplating the practice problem to clarify basic design principles needed for your research (phase one) informed by, for instance, the following sub-questions:

What are the current standard practices for addressing the needs of patients suffering from dementia?

What are the potential opportunities for more active engagement of the health care team in addressing the needs of patients suffering from dementia?

What attitudes and behavioral changes are required from the health care team to more actively address the needs of patients suffering from dementia?

Answering those sub-questions helps you prepare for a new set of questions focused on developing, testing, evaluating, and adapting an intervention, which is related to phase two of design research (chapter 7). A few examples of phase-two questions are:

What would be the design principles/components of a promising intervention?

What theoretical concept has informed the development of the intervention?

How effective is the intervention in practice?

How should the intervention be adapted based on pilot test results?

Exercise 6. Identify Sub-Questions (see page 91)

3.6. Guidelines for Drafting and Evaluating Practitioner Research Questions

As already stated, practitioner research is guided by the main research question and its sub-questions. Together they help you understand critical components of the practice problem that need clarification and determine the type of research you will be conducting. Therefore, it is very important for you to share and discuss your research questions with others (e.g., colleagues, members of the target groups, supervisors). In this section, you learn how to state and evaluate the significance and validity of your questions through a step-by-step process presented in the following 10 guidelines. Guidelines 1–9 are applicable to both main research questions and sub-questions. Guideline 10 specifically explains the relationship between the main question and the sub-questions.

Guideline 1: State It as a Question

Example. I want to confirm through practitioner research that the boys in my counseling sessions are more sensitive to peer pressure than the girls.

The problem with this example statement is the level of certainty that you indicate about knowing that boys are more sensitive to peer pressure. As discussed in chapter 1, adopting an inquisitive mind-set is the first critical step for conducting practitioner research. That means you need a main question regarding your practice problem that is stated as a question, so you can search for the answer and address the problem. In searching for the answer, however, you can clarify your assumptions in the form of different hypotheses and see if they are true or false after analyzing the data. Examples of better research questions in this case could be:

What kind of peer pressure have my students experienced?

How sensitive are the boys to peer pressure compared to the girls?

How does peer pressure affect boys and girls according to their own perspectives?

Guideline 2: Ask Open-Ended Questions

Example. Is an ankle bracelet a suitable device for keeping offenders in their houses and reducing the cost of incarceration?

In academic research, scientists often use closed-ended questions that can only be answered with a simple yes or no response when they want, for example, to test the effectiveness of a new medication in treating patients compared to no treatment. In practitioner research, however, almost always you need more than a yes or no response; solving a practice problem requires a great deal of details about context and processes. Hence, you need to ask questions that are open-ended, with interrogative words such as "what," "who," "when," "why," "where," "which," "how," and "to what extent." An example of a revised research question in this case could be:

To what extent is an ankle bracelet practical and effective in keeping offenders in their houses and reducing the costs of incarceration?

Guideline 3: Clearly State the Key Concepts of the Questions

Example. Which treatment plans work best for patients suffering from major depression?

In this case, the terms "treatment plans" and "work best" are not clearly defined and are open for interpretation. For example, medications, psychotherapy, and social support could all be considered treatment plans, although their intended outcomes and their mechanisms of effectiveness differ widely. Specifying the type of treatment plan can reduce the ambiguity in this example and point to specific intended outcomes in your research statement. When possible, it's better to refer to the body of literature and use standard terminology to clarify your key concepts. Furthermore, adding specific terms about the context of your research can further clarify the type and scope of your research and its intended outcomes. Examples of revised research questions in this case could be:

How satisfied are the patients diagnosed with major depression with the "atmosphere" of counseling sessions offered in our clinic?

How satisfied with the counseling sessions are patients' friends and family members who are engaged in "informal care"?

Here you can learn from the following two examples how to define the terms "atmosphere" and "informal care" in less ambiguous ways.

Example 1. "Atmosphere" in the context of my research means

- the climate is supportive;
- counselors and patients are interested and actively engaged in the process;
- patients express their views about the content of the program;
- patients report being comfortable in this group; and
- counselors and patients follow the agreed upon treatment plan and participate in all activities.

Example 2. I adhere to the following definition of informal care: "Formal care for older people usually refers to paid care services provided by a health care institution or individual for a person in need. Informal care refers to unpaid care provided by family, close relatives, friends, and neighbors. Both forms of caregiving involve a spectrum of tasks, but informal caregivers seldom receive enough training for these tasks. Formal caregivers are trained in the field, but the depth and quality of their training varies" (Li & Song, 2019).

Guideline 4: Be Attentive to Questions That Consist of More Than One Question

Example. What problems do children with fear of failure experience regarding self-determination, and can counseling help address the problems?

This example question is actually composed of two questions. The first question is about exploring the problems children have experienced, while the second question is about addressing the problems through counseling. Stating each question simply is very important and can make them easier to answer.

It would be better to break down the question and start with the following:

What problems do children with fear of failure experience regarding self-determination?

And only after answering this question would you ask the next question:

How can the problems that children with fear of failure experience regarding self-determination best be addressed?

Only combine questions if they are closely related and cannot lead to confusion:

Example. What are the pros and what are the cons of care robots for clients with intellectual disabilities?

Guideline 5: Do Not Ask Obvious Questions

Example. What are the routes of transmission for hospital-acquired (nosocomial) infections?

This question can be answered by reviewing the literature and reading relevant textbooks. Therefore, you wouldn't need practitioner research for this question. However, the question can be revised to focus on specific unknown aspects of this subject relevant to the context of a local hospital. Examples of revised questions for this case are:

To what extent are nosocomial infection prevention protocols followed in my hospital?

How can preventive measures against nosocomial infection be further improved?

Guideline 6: Do Not Make Assumptions Without Verification

Example. What were reasons for the success of cognitive behavioral therapy (CBT) in Detroit community health centers?

In this example, CBT is already introduced as a successful intervention without any further clarification or evidence. It is possible that after evaluating the services, the implementation of CBT is found to be successful according to specific criteria. But in this case, any claims like this should be backed by evidence and data. An example of a revised research question without nonverified assumptions is the following:

What are the opinions of clinical psychologists about the effectiveness of CBT counseling sessions offered in their health center?

Guideline 7: Substantiate Your Assumptions

Example. What are effective parent education and outreach strategies to achieve a 20 percent increase in the human papilloma virus (HPV) vaccination rate among 11- to 12-year-old students in Cleveland public middle schools?

This question is based on an assumption that parent education and outreach activities could potentially result in a 20 percent increase in the HPV vaccination rate among the target group of students. Such an assumption should be substantiated based on evidence, including professional experience. In addition, you would need to present data on the current rates of vaccination among your target group to better clarify the scope of work needed to answer the question. If you are able to substantiate your assumptions, then your question is a good one in its current form. If not, you will need to revise the statement.

Guideline 8: Ask Questions That Are Acceptable

Example. Which forms of parental corporal punishment produce better behavioral outcomes among preschool children?

A question like this is wrong for several reasons. First, according to the literature, physical punishment is not considered an appropriate disciplinary action; it can have severe, negative consequences for children's self-image and self-confidence. Second, the question indicates an assumption about the effectiveness of corporal punishment, despite valid counter arguments about ethical concerns related to this form of discipline. As a result, an unacceptable question like this is highly controversial, which compromises its potential to solve a practice problem or generate the required support for conducting this line of inquiry. Revised questions on this topic could include the following:

How do the parents participating in a parent education program discipline their preschool kids?

How effective are these actions?

How can the information gained by this research inform the design of a better parent education program?

Guideline 9: Ask Questions with Obvious Benefits for Others

Example. How can we enhance both the quality of clinical services provided by the health care team and the use of modern health information technology?

This question is relevant to most clinics because it is aligned with what patients, the community at large, funding agencies, and clinic leadership expect from health care centers. However, it is possible that a practitioner who is already overworked and underpaid may perceive a question like this as more work without enough reward. Such an attitude can serve as a major barrier—often not explicitly mentioned—to the success of your practitioner research study. Most of the time, however, you can shift the impact of such a question from being negative to positive by changing the wording, so the benefits of the research are more obvious. A good research question is one that both motivates and challenges you—as well as others—to unearth the answer. Therefore, the statement must be aligned with the organization's mission and it should sound beneficial and motivating to you, your colleagues, and your target groups. A revised statement with more explicit benefits for others is:

What ideas do health care practitioners have about how health information technology can improve the quality of services while benefiting various stakeholders in a health care center?

Guideline 10: Ask Sub-Questions That Contribute to Answering the Main Question

As mentioned in section 3.5, the combined answers to all of your sub-questions should provide you with what you need to answer your main question. In the following example, the first three questions are contributing to answering the main question, while question four is not relevant.

Example. What are the common approaches used by mental health practitioners working at the local hospital to diagnose and treat patients with frequent panic and anxiety attacks?

What are the diagnostic methods for identification and classification of panic and anxiety attack disorders according to the literature?

What methods are used by the practitioners of the local hospital during the diagnostic phase?

What kind of treatment approaches are used by the practitioners for treating patients with panic and anxiety attack disorders?

What are the comparative effects of the employed diagnostic and treatment approaches?

Exercise 7. Evaluating Research Questions (see page 91)

3.7. Documenting Your Findings

Documentation is an important aspect of practitioner research in every stage. Here we will provide you with a simple checklist of a few important steps to make sure that you have documented everything after completing the focusing stage and discussing the results. While going through such documentation, you may need to revise your practice problem, which can subsequently change other requirements, such as the need for additional orientation activities. This illustrates (again) the iterative nature of conducting practitioner research. Later, you will use your notes to integrate the findings into part C of the research plan, which will be discussed in the next chapter.

Documentation Checklist

☐ *Literature review*
Prepare a comprehensive description of the practice problem based on the literature. Highlight the standard definitions and description of the main aspects of the practice problem, possible solutions, any key components and sub-components, and interactions between them, according to reliable sources of information.

☐ *Research objective*
Write down the final version of your research objective and the significance of the objective for the professional practice, your organization, and yourself.

☐ *Research question*
Write down the final version of the main question and the sub-questions as well as their corresponding key components.

☐ *Practice problem*
Update, redefine, and revise the first description of your practice problem.

3.8. Summary

Activities that you do during the focusing stage guide you through developing a deeper understanding of the practice problem, which is informed by the published literature and professional knowledge. This is mainly achieved by doing an in-depth problem analysis based on a plausible theoretical framework. In this stage, you move beyond the literature search and engage in critically reading, reflecting, summarizing, and synthesizing information gained from relevant and valid sources of your choosing. A structured literature review helps you better describe and define the practice problem by learning from previous researchers' experiences and other sources and comparing them with your own description of the practice problem in your professional practice. This can further enrich your problem analysis and gives you better insight into what additional knowledge you need to acquire.

The next logical step of the focusing stage, after conducting the literature review and problem analysis, is identifying and stating your research objectives and questions, which will serve as the guiding theme of your practitioner research study. The research objective indicates what you aim to learn and/or improve throughout your research. The research question is derived from the research objective to clarify what we don't know and guide appropriate study designs to answering the questions. Five basic types of research questions are descriptive, defining, comparative, evaluative, and explanatory, and there are a variety of techniques that you can use for identifying and selecting relevant questions and sub-questions that are aligned with your research objective. By clarifying what is possible within a set time frame and with existing resources, the scope of the research can be determined. To make the research more focused and organized, the main question can be broken down into sub-questions in a way that the cumulative answers to the sub-questions provide you with what you need to answer the respective main question. Ten guidelines were introduced to help you assess the validity of the main question and sub-questions. Lastly, a simple checklist can be used to better organize and document your findings after completing the focusing stage and sharing the results.

Exercise 1. Searching the Literature: Finding Useful Textual Sources

The purpose of this exercise is to practice the processes of finding relevant textual sources and evaluating their usefulness. This exercise is most suitable to be conducted in a group.

> Your organization has requested the staff to investigate appropriate in-service training to prepare the staff to deal with client conflicts involving aggressive behaviors.

Each member of the group is tasked with finding at least two sources relevant to conflict management and aggressive behaviors in health care and social service settings. Each member of the team will evaluate the credibility of the sources found by another member (based on the criteria presented in the appendix). Share and discuss your findings in the group and compile a list of the most reliable sources for this topic.

Exercise 2. Prepare for the Literature Review: Link the Concepts with Sources

This exercise helps you identify links between different textual sources and the research subject. This exercise works best if performed as a group.

Each member of the group will select a source relevant to the chosen topic. Discuss with the group any connections you find between the source and the topic of interest. Then clarify any commonalities and differences between your selected sources while trying to find explanations for any differences you have found.

Exercise 3. Research Objectives

When you draft a research objective, it is important to determine if it is directly or indirectly aligned with your organization's vision and mission. After reading the following scenarios, state the possible benefits of such inquiries for their respective organizations.

> Frank is a full-time employee at a local social service agency. He loves sports and has a busy social life. In addition, he is in the process of setting up his own business. He is getting overwhelmed and needs to do a better job managing his time. Frank wants to plan his free time and his life-related activities to lower his work-related stress and to be successful both personally and professionally.

> Jasmine loves cooking and she writes cookbooks in her free time. Her current project is a cookbook that focuses on healthy food for seniors according to their taste preferences. She works in a nursing home and she wants to set up a small-scale research project in which she can interview the residents to learn about their favorite recipes and their dietary restrictions.

Exercise 4. Main Research Questions

Five techniques were introduced for identifying suitable research questions (section 3.3). Put one or two of these techniques into practice based on any actual or fictional practice problem you choose. Discuss the results and whatever you learn through the process with other members of your group or organization.

Exercise 5. Determine the Scope of a Research Question

Two techniques for determining the scope of your research question were provided (section 3.4). Practice both techniques with example questions from technique 4 (section 3.3) and discuss your findings with your fellow students or colleagues.

Exercise 6. Identify Sub-Questions

In technique 4 (section 3.3), several examples are provided for different types of research questions. Choose one or two questions from the list and come up with four to six relevant sub-questions. This exercise works best if performed as a group. Review the results based on the instructions described in the guidelines found in section 3.6.

Exercise 7. Evaluating Research Questions

Team up with a peer or buddy and discuss why the following research questions are not properly stated.

1. How can I improve a trusting relationship between my clients by having them work with another peer?
2. Why do so few women choose careers in construction management?
3. Why is this organization not sufficiently staffed to implement the results of the client satisfaction surveys and improve the quality of services?
4. What is the process for actively engaging external consultants in addressing the problems and planning the training activities of the agency staff?
5. What are ways to prepare students from underrepresented minority backgrounds to minimize their chances of academic failure?
6. What are common problems faced by new foster parents in fulfilling their obligations and how can keeping a journal help?
7. Has the sex education program offered to 12- to 14-year-old middle school students of the City of Los Angeles reduced the number of teen pregnancies?

REFERENCE

Li, J. & Song, Y. (2019). Formal and informal care. In D. Gu & M. Dupre (Eds.), *Encyclopedia of Gerontology and Population Aging* (online), Springer. https://doi.org/10.1007/978-3-319 -69892-2_847-1

4

Planning

In chapters 2 and 3 you learned how to conduct a thorough problem analysis and develop useful objectives and questions for your practitioner research study. Now you are ready to work on your research plan, which is about describing and planning the activities needed for conducting the study (figure 4.1). Such activities can include collecting and analyzing data, drawing conclusions, designing innovative interventions, documenting methods, and developing strategies for dissemination.

In this chapter, you will learn about data collection tools that you can use—or develop, if not available—in practitioner research. First, you will be introduced to the questions that can help you choose suitable data collection methods. Then, the main methods for data collection are discussed, along with other alternatives. The process of how to identify research participants and estimate the number of needed respondents is described. You will then be shown how to prepare an effective work plan for research activities. The standard format and criteria for structuring a comprehensive research plan, along with assessing the cohesiveness of the structure are presented. Chapter 4 concludes with a brief summary of the discussions and relevant exercises.

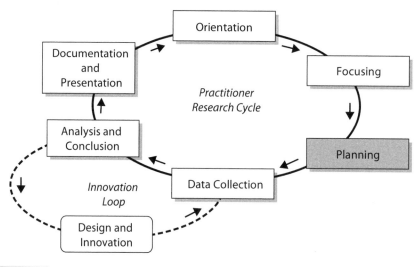

Figure 4.1

Key component of practitioner research: Planning

4.1. Selecting Data Collection Methods

You collect a lot of data as part of your daily activities as a health care or social service practitioner. You attend professional meetings, speak with your colleagues, share your expert opinions and get feedback, observe your clients/patients, read emails and other pertinent documents, and participate in professional development activities. As a result, you acquire and use a substantial amount of work-related data in order to function as a high-impact practitioner. However, much of this valuable data is often underutilized due to memory loss, poor documentation, or less than optimal data management practices. Therefore, practitioners often may not have the information they need when they need it. Practitioner research helps you to become more organized and systematic in collecting data from multiple sources, and in verifying the data's credibility. If done correctly, you will end up with structured qualitative and quantitative datasets that can be analyzed to answer your research questions.

There are multiple data collection methods, and each is suitable for answering specific types of questions while possessing unique strengths and limitations. You need to decide which methods are most appropriate for answering your research questions. Practitioners often use more than one method to maximize the overall strength, validity, and reliability of their data through triangulation (see section 1.4). For example, if you are interested in finding out about a typical day of a homeless person in your city, one way of collecting data is to spend a few days observing homeless individuals in a local shelter and/or in the community. Another option is to interview a few homeless individuals about their daily activities. Furthermore, you can visit a shelter or a soup kitchen to conduct focus group discussions, asking the participants about what they usually do in a typical day.

The following four questions can help you choose the most relevant data collection methods for answering your questions.

To What Degree Does the Data Collection Method Contribute to Answering the Research Question?

As a general rule, selecting a data collection method is based on its ability to generate the data needed to answer your questions. In most cases, you need to employ multiple methods to generate sufficient information.

Example. An oncology nurse wants to conduct a study to answer the following question: What psychological support services can improve oncology patients' quality of life at home? She starts by reviewing the hospital's policy and procedures as well as the psychological support offered prior, during, and after treatment. Then she decides to conduct individual in-depth interviews with her psychology and social work colleagues to assess whether the patients receive enough emotional and psychological support while in the hospital. Furthermore, she wants to know what her colleagues think about the impact of such services on patients' ability to deal with challenges they usually face at home posttreatment.

In this example, the oncology nurse wants to understand the impact of psychological support services offered in the hospital on patients' quality of life. In order to acquire a more comprehensive answer, she needs to understand her patients' challenges and difficulties after the completion of the treatment as well as their perceptions about the quality of services and their desired living standards. Therefore, in addition to interviewing her colleagues, she needs to interview the patients or have them complete a questionnaire to determine whether the services have been comprehensive and effective according to their expectations. In this example, you can clearly see that certain methods can partly contribute to answering a question while not providing the full answer.

Is the Selected Method the Best Possible Option for Answering the Question?

It is usually more efficient to use methods, tools, and resources that are already available and accessible to practitioners in a professional practice setting to answer research questions. It is important to carefully examine and evaluate the credibility and cost effectiveness of the methods you propose to use (see section 4.2 for more details).

Example. You are an undergraduate student majoring in social work who is required to do research to assess and compare possible career and graduate studies opportunities relevant to your field. Your preferred method is to interview a few graduates and senior practitioners to learn about the available opportunities, including their advantages, disadvantages, costs, and benefits.

Conducting individual interviews makes sense and could potentially provide answers to your research question. It is, however, very important to determine whether this is the most efficient method. In this example, you might be able to answer your research question by first visiting your university's center for graduate school and career development, if one exists, where you would be able to discuss your research question with the staff and get ideas about relevant resources to read and key informants to interview. It is more efficient to get the introductory information by reviewing textual sources and online profiles of your key informants and then writing down relevant questions to ask each person rather than interviewing a few random individuals using one set of questions.

Has the Data Been Validated through Triangulation?

As discussed in chapter 1, triangulation—using multiple sources, methods, and researchers—is a powerful approach for verifying and validating data (see section 1.4, guideline 1). We can better trust answers that are based on validated data acquired from more than one source (e.g., colleagues, patients, senior experts) through complementary methods (e.g., quantitative, qualitative) and by a team of researchers from diverse background (e.g., nursing, psychology, social work). In practitioner research, you want to make sure that you utilize methods with the potential to cover more than one dimension or perspective related to the practice problem.

Example. The board of trustees of a psychiatric hospital has announced a master plan that includes enhancing the quality of nursing care based on a vision and a set of values embraced by all stakeholders. A nurse practitioner wants to conduct a study to identify and clarify the core values and concepts that the nursing department finds most relevant and critical. She plans to review current policy guidelines and case studies to ensure that the core values are aligned with recommended procedures and best practices. The vision and the core values will ultimately guide efforts over the next few years to improve the quality of care and enhance the capacity of the nursing department.

In this example, getting the information from the nursing department's providers and administrative staff is a good way to obtain insights and make conclusions about a set of core values. In addition, the nurse practitioner will review sources from published literature and policy guidelines that could help her triangulate the information gained from the interviews. However, there are other potential sources that need to be captured, which could bring different perspectives about nursing care standards and core values perceived by patients, family members, funders, and partner organizations. Capturing such input through different methods (e.g., focus group discussions, surveys, individual interviews) and by engaging researchers from other disciplines (e.g., psychiatrists, social workers, psychologists) can provide more comprehensive information and ample opportunities to determine the most valid set of values through triangulation. Even when collecting input from patients and family members, several complementary methods could be used, such as reviewing new patients' intake files, listening to and documenting patients' needs and concerns at the time of admission, conducting exit interviews with family members, and so on. The process can help you form a valid impression about patients' real needs, available nursing care practices, and a set of core values attached to ideal services.

Is the Data Collection Method a Good Fit for the Type of Sub-Question?

As discussed in chapter 1, there are different types of research questions and sub-questions: descriptive, defining, comparative, evaluative, and explanatory. We also learned that each sub-question focuses on answering a specific part of the main research question so that the sum of the answers to all sub-questions should provide the full answer to the main question. Therefore, it's common to have a main question of a certain type (e.g., evaluative) with various types of sub-questions (e.g., descriptive, comparative, or explanatory). In this case, you need to make sure to choose methods that are a good fit for each type of sub-question.

Exercise 1. Evaluating Selected Data Collection Method(s) (see page 117)

Exercise 2. Generating a Client/Patient Summary Report (see page 117)

4.2. Data Collection Methods

Data collection methods can be either quantitative or qualitative. *Quantitative methods* are used to collect statistically measurable data through polls, questionnaires, surveys, or analyzing preexisting data for a new purpose. Quantitative data are in the form of numbers, and they are often presented in tables, graphs, and charts. They are analyzed to either describe certain properties (e.g., frequency, rate, proportion, average) or compare differences between various groups in order to test a hypothesis. You often collect quantifiable data from a smaller sample of participants to better understand and generalize it to a larger group. In some practitioner research studies, you may need to employ standard research methodologies for calculating your sample size and making sure that it represents the larger group. Such methodological details are not the focus of this book and can be found in research-methods textbooks. In most cases, however, you would be able to answer your research questions through simple methodologies described here and in the following chapters. Questions and tools used in quantitative methods are often standardized and tested for validity and reliability, so they can be better trusted when used in various situations with different participants. For example, respondents are given identical questions with predefined response options or they are observed based on a structured checklist. Such responses are aggregated and converted into numbers (quantified).

Qualitative methods of data collection provide information about context and subjective views of life experience that in its original form cannot be expressed numerically or analyzed statistically. For example, when data from a patient satisfaction survey are quantified into being satisfied or not satisfied, you will end up with a hard number that doesn't provide much insight on how and why the patients experience a service a certain way. In general, qualitative data is textual information (in the form of interview transcripts, observation reports, and notes taken from textual sources) or an auditory and/or a visual representation (film, picture, or other medium). In other words, you may also collect visual or auditory qualitative data that later can be analyzed and transformed into textual or even numerical presentations. Qualitative questions are more open-ended in nature, allowing respondents to freely share their experiences, opinions, and knowledge. In this context, "open-ended" means that response options for the questions are not predefined. Qualitative questions are often stated with exploratory phrases that allow long answers and use probing guides to solicit more details. Respondents are encouraged to answer the questions in their own words, and everything is often transcribed verbatim.

Practitioner researchers often choose to use both quantitative and qualitative methods—so-called *mixed-method studies*—to better understand the scope of the practice problem, contributing factors, and possible solutions. Mixed-method studies take advantage of the strengths of both qualitative and quantitative data.

The main types of data collection are document analysis, systematic observation, interviewing, surveying, testing, alternative methods, and site visits.

Document Analysis

In health care and social services settings, in addition to scientific and professional sources, other documents and client records can be used for data collection, such as standard operating procedures, patient/client files, meeting notes, organization policy documents, handbooks, and special reports (e.g., quality improvement, evaluation, annual report). These sources contain retrospective data that have already been collected. Documents such as patient records, inventories, and reports can be used as primary or secondary sources of data to answer the research questions. Documents such as meeting notes and case reports often contain qualitative information about the context and nature of the practice problem, stakeholders' perceptions, and the results of past responses to the problem. Further, you can use internal sources of information to learn more about the organizational culture, terminology, and policies.

> *Example.* Kim is working in a nursing home where most residents have expressed loneliness and boredom. She conducted a literature review to better understand the practice problem and social activities that could potentially address the problem. She learned about the common emotional needs of the residents while transitioning from being independent to depending on others. She makes a list of potential activities that could meet such needs and protect the residents from being depressed, such as special celebrations, book clubs, musical events, outdoor activities, social groups, and religious services. Next, she contacts the recreational department where she gains access to internal documents such as the nursing home calendar, meeting notes, and evaluation reports. She intends to use these documents to collect both quantitative and qualitative data on the type of social events, the frequency of each event, level of attendance, and overall quality and effectiveness of the current recreational programs. This will give Kim a better idea of how to improve current services to address the practice problem.

In this example, Kim studies relevant literature to corroborate, and possibly explain, her practical observations. The results of her practitioner research study could lead to recommendations for improving recreational services based on scientific evidence and professional retrospective data resulting from document analysis.

Important Tips

- The strength of document analysis depends on the quality of the professional records: both internal procedures for collecting professional information and organizational policies for documenting and organizing such information. You might not get everything you need from analyzing available documents, and therefore you may still need to collect prospective data to fully answer your research questions.
- Make sure that you obtain all required authorizations and necessary approvals from management (and if applicable, relevant ethics committees) when using clients' record and other private/confidential information.

- Always be mindful of potential biases resulting from individual preferences by critically reviewing documents produced by different individuals. For instance, meeting notes could be drafted mainly from a notetaker's perspective on the matter and might not accurately reflect the discussions and conclusions. Also, practitioners can vary widely in how they document their work in patient/client records.

Systematic Observation

Observation is one of the most readily available strategies for collecting important quantitative and qualitative data relevant to a practice problem. As a practitioner researcher, there are many important things that you observe and consider every day.

They could be observations directly related to your professional practice or positive and negative events related to the context of your practice. You can gain significant insights into your practice problem and collect valuable data needed to answer your questions by making well-planned systematic observations using tools such as checklists, charts, notebooks, calendars, and journals. For example, you can use a checklist to document how well nursing students measure patients' blood pressure or observe a training session to assess qualitatively the level of interactions between the students and the instructor. Some other examples of situations where you can make systematic observations include patients working together in group therapy, colleagues' reactions in a meeting, patients' posture while lifting weights in a physical therapy session, children playing games on the playground, or a video recorded in a homeless shelter. A quantitative approach is relevant when you are interested in documenting quantifiable events and steps, while qualitative observation is used when you are interested in understanding how and why certain things happen.

Example. A supervising nurse in a prenatal care unit decides to use systematic observation to conduct research to improve the quality and effectiveness of services. He wants to check the inventory of the medications, supplies, and equipment to assess the sufficiency of resources. He prepares a list of every needed resource with empty boxes in front of each item for writing down their quantities. He also creates a checklist based on expected quality standards for evaluating, educating, and providing health care services to the clients. After obtaining needed permissions, he will observe a few nurses while they provide services using his checklist, and he will make notes about their level of adherence to the standard protocols.

The above example shows how systematic observation can be used to turn important insights into daily practice.

Important Tips

- Observation requires thorough preparation. You need to make decisions beforehand about your purpose, what you intend to observe, tools required for collecting and documenting data, and the application of your findings.

Direct observations are often converted into notes, checklists, or audio file transcriptions.

- Using systematic observation as a data collection method has important strengths (e.g., developing a clearer understanding of the problem in real time) and important weaknesses (e.g., filtering or amplifying certain realities based on your individual preference). We recommend that you be fully informed about potential strengths and weaknesses and try to stay as neutral and free of bias as possible.

- One limitation is that rare events such as patients' reactions to a unique situation are difficult to capture by this method.

- Observation often comes with the price of changing the natural dynamics of professional practice as the result of your being there and watching and/or recording the goings on. You can often mitigate this limitation by observing as remotely and seamlessly as possible and communicating clearly the purpose of your observation, while asking for permission beforehand.

- When observation is done by more than one person, make sure that the process, the tools, and the collected data are pilot-tested and compared so that any discrepancies are identified and resolved. This is to ensure that your whole team uses this method and collects data as consistently and systematically as possible.

Interviewing, Surveying, and Testing

This section presents a number of data collection methods aimed at assessing participants' attitudes, behaviors, knowledge, skills, and/or competencies in various situations. Participants often report their observations, thoughts, and ideas or share what they know. In other words, interviewing, surveying, and testing are methods used to view or perceive the world through the eyes and minds of the participants. Sometimes the questions intend to reveal facts, such as participants' sociodemographic, familial, and environmental characteristics. In other cases, participants' feelings, perceptions, and interpretations are at the center of attention. In testing, the focus is on knowledge, skills, and competencies. Interviewing, surveying, and testing can be done through quantitative and qualitative methods.

Qualitative methods vary, but some commonly used methods are brainstorming with patients on a simple question while they are receiving their treatment, conducting focus groups and key informant interviews, and soliciting and reviewing anonymous comments dropped in a box.

Examples of quantitative methods include patients' intake interviews using a questionnaire, polls, self-administered posttreatment exit surveys, standardized tests (e.g., depression, anxiety, perceived social support), and program evaluation assessments.

Example. A group of youth counselors, who work at inner city high schools to assist students dealing with substance abuse, get together for a monthly meeting. The leader of the group notices that most counselors have trouble working with the new information technology and registration systems. She decides to conduct a brainstorming session to better understand the problem. Later, she meets with a few counselors to conduct in-depth interviews to better understand their perceptions of the problem, its main causes, and potential solutions. Lastly, the team leader creates a questionnaire based on the acquired information to be filled out by all youth counselors to explain how they use the system and what problems they experience.

In this example, the team leader wants to understand and address the problem using qualitative methods followed by a quantitative survey using a self-administered questionnaire. This will help the team leader to more thoroughly understand the problem from the counselors' perspective and to use their ideas and recommendations to help address the problem.

Testing can be used as a method to assess the knowledge, skills, and competencies of study participants. For example, *pre-post testing* (surveying participants before and after an intervention, such as a class) is a convenient way of measuring how much they have learned. Educational and training modules often have question sets that can be used for designing relevant tests. Just bear in mind that certain tests, especially those conducted with minors, require informed consent and/or permission from the participants and their legal guardians.

Example. John is an educator interested in testing a hypothesis on whether engagement in some sort of physical activity (such as throwing and catching a ball) can enhance the effectiveness and retention of information in a math education program. To do so, he designed a study to test the effectiveness of practicing multiplication tables while performing a physical exercise (the *intervention group*). To assess the effect of the intervention, John compares the results with another group of students who practice multiplication tables without engaging in any physical activities (the *control group*). Both intervention and control groups take a knowledge test immediately afterward and two weeks after the training.

The timing of data collection may play an important role in how participants respond and may affect the results. This can be due to such issues as important co-occurring events, the political climate, personal problems, or macroeconomic issues. Such factors may affect individuals' overall willingness to participate in your research.

Example. The employees of a community hospital are interviewed about their job satisfaction and motivation to work shortly after attending a meeting where a major budget cut and a plan for layoffs is announced.

Interviews, surveys and tests, like observations, may be conducted more than one time depending on the research question. If you intend to document patients' experiences with a new treatment method in various phases, you may need to interview them at different time periods. However, if you just want to assess the patients' experience during the first phase of the treatment, a one-time interview or survey should be enough.

The context in which the questions are asked may influence the answers. For example, if members of a community suspect that your research could result in bad publicity for their neighborhood, they may decide not to reveal everything. Or if a self-administered questionnaire designed to assess the performance of health care center employees is not anonymous and might be used for annual reviews, the employees may not be entirely truthful or forthcoming in their answers.

Important Tips

- Interviewing, surveying, and testing are founded on asking questions, which means you often rely on subjective answers reported by your participants that cannot be easily verified or validated through other measures.

- You can use interviewing, surveying, and testing to obtain information relevant to your practice problem. Remember that the questions determine which topics are covered and what kind of data are generated. It is always recommended to revise and validate your questions to make sure that you are getting what you need. Some questions often contain terms that are ambiguous and thus open to different interpretation by participants. People usually react differently when encountering such terms as "patient-centered," "self-reliant," "interactive," "outcome-oriented," "evidence-based," "transparency," "patient participation," "appropriate level of care," "compliance," "risk management," and so on. Similar problems may arise with such words as "much" or "many," "good" or "bad," "few" or "little," "simple" or "difficult." You need to be aware of such problems and always consider what the terms used can mean in the context in which you are collecting your data. In order to reduce the chances of being misunderstood, potentially ambiguous terms need to be clearly defined.

- Be as clear as possible about how you intend to document and organize your data. For example, are you going to audio record your individual in-depth interviews and transcribe them? How will you store the information? Do you intend to use qualitative analysis software or organize the notes manually? Having detailed plans and protocols for acquiring, documenting, aggregating, and organizing your data will make your practitioner research more robust and rigorous.

- Even when preferred, it is sometimes difficult to conduct face-to-face interviews due to logistical/technical challenges and time constraints. Alternative methods for collecting information can be through phone interviews, online surveys, or onsite surveys using self-administered questionnaires.

- Surveying and testing are relatively easy methods to collect large amounts of information in a short period of time that otherwise would be hard to obtain. Less-structured questions are usually more flexible, and more answers could be regarded as relevant to such questions. On the other hand, answers to more-structured questions are limited to fewer predefined options. One advantage of working with more-structured data is that they are relatively easy to analyze. However, participants have fewer opportunities to elaborate on highly structured questions and thus may not fully express the reality behind certain topics or questions.

- Group discussions are effective ways for acquiring in-depth answers to research questions, as members' interactions often spark new ideas and enhance participants' willingness to share more details. However, while it is beneficial to facilitate group discussions, not all participants may be comfortable speaking freely in front of others, especially if it involves discussing confidential or sensitive issues.

Alternative Methods

Alternative methods refer to a class of nonconventional data collection strategies that include such things as storytelling, role-playing, visualization, photography, and the like. Such methods are often developed to bring participants together in familiar places and help them contribute to the research in ways that are more in tune with their own life experiences. Sometimes alternative methods are used in tandem with conventional methods such as document analysis, systematic observations, interviewing, surveying, and testing but with more flexibility and attention to the contextual characteristics of the setting. In chapter 5, you will learn more about seven categories of alternative methods: expressive, visual, narrative, creative thinking and writing, decision-making and valuation, measuring, and social experiments. Here we provide a brief description and representative example of each.

Expressive Methods

Such methods are used to help participants express their lived experiences and knowledge through engagement in activities such as role-playing, participatory drama, and other performing arts. For example, participants are given case scenarios and asked to express themselves through the eyes of their fictitious characters.

Visual Methods

Depending on the subject, some participants may find using cameras, drawings, and visual conceptualization techniques more powerful to communicate the realities of their daily struggles rather than saying them in words. For example, middle school students are asked to take photographs of their own community problems and explain why they took the photos. This is called photovoice, a powerful alternative method for visualizing, discussing, and addressing the issues. Such techniques based on visual or participatory content encourage participants to express themselves differently (Lorenz & Kolb, 2009; Packard, 2008; Von Unger, 2013).

Narrative Methods

You can use narrative techniques and stories in various ways to gain insight into respondents' experiences and/or their views about a particular topic (Bold, 2012; Ledwith & Springett, 2010; Van Biene et al., 2012). It may be easier for participants, such as those who are younger, to contribute their stories and engage in informal dialogues rather than responding to interview questions. For example, storytelling can be used as a method to gain insights into the practice problem either directly from the participant's perspective or indirectly through a fictitious story told about a third person.

Creative Thinking and Writing Methods

This category of alternative methods refers to such techniques as mind mapping and journaling that allows elaboration and reflection on participants' experiences and ideas. Reflection is a method that allows people to learn from their experience. These experiences include action aspects (acting), cognitive aspects (thinking), emotional aspects (feeling) and motivational aspects (willingness) (Geenen, 2017). Reflection is often an implicit or explicit part of the daily actions of professionals and clients. There are various reflection models and techniques that you can use to gain insight into (learning) experiences of yourself and others. For example, by asking participants to keep a prestructured journal, you can gain valuable insights into how and why certain activities are conducted.

Decision-Making and Valuation

You can acquire useful data through this category of methods while helping participants make important decisions related to a practice problem. Furthermore, participants can engage in valuating available factors and options through such techniques as nominal group discussion or the use of scorecards. For example, you present the participants with a specific statement and ask them to take a position for or against that statement. This type of activity can help them to more naturally express and discuss their views.

Measuring

Measurements are often taken in research with the aid of reliable tools and instruments. They are used, for instance, to help reach diagnoses or to evaluate various therapies. Measuring tools can be developed for physical examination, self-reports, function tests, and laboratory research. In practitioner research, you may find creative ways for measuring variables of interest in and/or outside of the practice setting. For example, you may ask your client to self-measure their blood pressure at home several times a day.

Social Experiments

Professional practice settings often provide opportunities for conducting novel, natural experiments. Such experiments can generate data that lead to improvement of services and/or set the stage for conducting more robust studies. For example, you can compare educational sessions offered for various target groups to find out how such programs should be tailored to meet the needs of specific groups of clients. However, you must always carefully consider and comply with the ethical issues related to conducting social experiments (see chapter 5).

Important Tips

- Obtaining research data from alternative methods often requires high levels of creativity. The data are often in formats that are not quite easy to use. We suggest that you spend enough time with your colleagues to develop novel approaches for collecting and analyzing data that can help answer your research question.

■ Alternative methods of data collection are often quite similar with activities and discussions that respondents have been engaged in within the context of day-to-day professional practice. Therefore, the respondents may not feel that they are participating in a study. However, you need to still explain the reason for engaging in such activities.

■ Many alternative methods of data collection intend to reach certain groups of people who traditionally are hard to reach. By using alternative methods, you give voice to those who are underrepresented and enhance the democratic and process validity of your research project.

■ Many alternative methods of data collection provide rich, qualitative data offering valuable insights into the experiences, perceptions, and opinions of the respondents. Therefore, the respondents often feel that they are being listened to, which can both increase the level of support for your research project and empower them to better contribute to their own health and well-being.

Site Visits

Visiting sites or participating in professional events can provide you with a unique opportunity to interact and speak with people, make important observations, and gain access to critical resources and documents. If done systematically, valuable data and insights can be obtained, for instance, by visiting a professional organization, attending a conference, dropping by other departments at your organization, or participating in a public event. The site visit is an important method of data collection in practitioner research that provides you with a unique opportunity to employ the previously discussed methods in a particular location, allowing you to both triangulate your data and to have firsthand experience with your subject of interest.

Every organization has a unique working environment, which is formally or informally formed around a combination of shared opinions, set routines, social agreements, and values. When collecting data through conventional methods, sometimes we "can't see the forest for the trees," meaning we are too involved in the details of a problem to look at the larger picture. At a site visit, you have the chance to experience complex phenomena as an integrated whole, while also having the opportunity to explore important details. In addition, visiting other organizations in your field can widen your perspective, as you see others approaching the same practice problems you experience in a different way. Site visits can be prompted by the need to gain access to expertise and capacities that don't exist in your own organization, or to find out firsthand how others deal with issues you often face. Therefore, visiting other organizations can greatly help you to learn how they operate, share information, make improvements, and address common practice problems.

Example. Sharon is a case manager at a drug recovery center. She is working on a research project to understand effective ways of getting physicians, psychologists, and social workers to communicate with each other on matters related to patients' individual treatment needs. As an initial step, she decides to visit a well-known local drug recovery center and learn from their experience.

Important Tips

- Site visits give you the opportunity to combine other data collection methods, such as document analysis, observation, and interviewing. But you need to be well prepared and organized to get the most out of the site visit. For example, you will be far more successful in reaching your goals by making simple preparations, such as creating a list of documents to review, identifying areas of interest or daily routines to observe, and preparing questions to ask specific stakeholders, experts, and participants.

- Preparing for site visits requires careful planning that takes time. Make sure that you prepare a detailed plan for your site visit, share your plan with others and make changes based on their feedback. Let your research questions guide your planning process and the frequency of your visits.

- Internal site visits can also be useful, providing insight into parts of your organization that you wouldn't otherwise be able to obtain. Some examples are visiting sites or departments other than yours, shadowing an expert, or attending certain meetings for the first time.

- You are encouraged to involve other colleagues in site visits and turn it into a group activity. Cohesive teams are usually more successful in obtaining high quality data, mainly due to the interactions between the members that provide the opportunity for the integration of multiple perspectives.

- Consider inviting someone from the site you visit to come to your organization in order to create more opportunities for in-depth learning and exchange of information.

- Not every organization welcomes external visitors or systematic information gathering. This can be due to concerns about losing their competitive edge, revealing proprietary information, fearing negative publicity, or exposing sensitive data. Do not assume all organizations will want to host you. Take time to contact the organization, explain the nature of your intended visit, and share details about how you intend to collect and use the data.

4.3. Participant Selection

In a practitioner research study, significant amounts of data are collected either from preexisting material (textual, visual, audio), individuals, or groups of participants in the context of professional practice. Each of the preexisting sources, persons, or groups from which you obtain data is called a *research unit*. During the planning phase, you need to make sure that your research units are identified and relevant arrangements are made for you to have appropriate and ethical access to the information. Allow enough time to make appointments and to obtain materials. Gaining access to people and material is often more time-consuming than you think.

As in other forms of research, you need to identify the group of people or materials from which you want to collect data. That group is your *target population*. In many cases, you don't have access to everyone (or everything) in that population. For example, when conducting research on client satisfaction in a counseling agency, you likely would not be able to interview all past and current clients due to their sheer number and your limited resources. In such cases you need to draw a *sample* from the population, that is, a manageable subgroup for your study. Your sample size depends on the size of the target population, the scope of your research, and practical considerations such as access and available resources. Sometimes practitioner research deals with a small target population (e.g., all members of a community outreach team). In this case, a practitioner may be able to collect data from all the team members. But if the target population is all social workers at a large social services agency, you need to select a sample that reflects the desired diversity of the entire group.

Your selection criteria will differ from one study to another, depending on what you identify as important characteristics of the members of the population. Commonly, you want to ensure diversity based on such factors as participants' sociodemographic characteristics, levels of experience, roles, and the like. In most practitioner research studies, you can use common sense to define the size and characteristics of your sample. In some situations, however, when the population of interest is too large (e.g., all patients receiving home care in a particular neighborhood) and you are testing a specific hypothesis, you need to draw a large enough sample that is representative of the entire population. A suitable *representative sample* is often drawn randomly and systematically using standard sampling techniques. In most practitioner research studies, however, the selection process relies on a logical justification to ensure that the size and composition of your sample is appropriate to your needs so that you will be able to generalize the findings to the target population with an acceptable level of certainty.

> *Example.* Raquel is working in a home care agency in Virginia. As a quality assurance expert, she is interested in conducting a postvisitation client satisfaction survey. Raquel decides to survey a subset of participants that is similar to the target population with respect to age, gender, health care needs, services received, the time of the visits, and the presence of a caregiver at home. This approach will help Raquel understand the overall perception of participants by surveying only a subset of the clients.

Representative samples can be identified in different ways. For large groups, the most frequently used method is *random* (or *probability*) *sampling*. This technique allows you to stay neutral and gives each member of the target population an equal chance of being selected. To apply this technique, you need a database of everyone's names with unique identification numbers linked to each name. Then, you pick your participants either through a lottery system or by using random numbers. You can find several free random number generators online. The selected individuals make up your sample population.

Example. Karen is a dietician facilitating a support group program for patients with eating disorders. She wants to understand the impact of the program on the participants' health behavior. To do so, she decides to interview a subset of 10 patients from the target population of 150. She creates a list of patients that is numbered from 1 to 150. She uses Google's random number generator to generate 10 numbers between 1 to 150. Each time she presses "generate," the system generates a number. She writes down the first 10 numbers and invites those individuals to participate in a group discussion.

When random sampling is not feasible, samples can be selected through nonprobability methods. Nonrandom selection can lower the representativeness of the sample, as participants' chances of being selected will not be equal. Therefore, the resulting sample could be influenced by various factors and conditions (Delnooz, 2010). However, through careful planning and selection, you can significantly enhance the similarity of the sample to the target population. A few examples of nonrandom sampling techniques are described next.

Convenience Sampling

Sometimes it is hard to reach the target population, especially when dealing with at-risk groups (e.g., homeless individuals, mental health patients, people living with HIV/AIDS). Through convenience sampling, you can recruit your participants from known places and communities, such as mental health clinics, homeless shelters, and the like. In this technique, you can enhance the relevance of the sample by selecting a larger number of individuals from different places or from a variety of days and times, thus increasing the diversity of the sample. You need to be careful not to include an individual more than once.

Snowball Sampling

The metaphor for this technique is a snowball rolling downhill and accumulating more snow along the way. When your target population is hard to reach, you could ask your initial research participants to help you recruit more (Goodman, 1961). At-risk populations with shared characteristics and professionals who serve them often interact with a larger group of hard-to-reach individuals. Through snowball sampling, you may be able to reach an otherwise hard-to-reach community (e.g., people with drug addiction) by starting with health care providers and their patients. In this case, the provider (your first point of contact) shares her professional experience and refers you to a few patients. After interviewing each new patient, your knowledge increases and you receive more referrals to other people with addiction from those whom you already interviewed. Depending on your practice problem, the first point of contact could be a program coordinator, another researcher, a colleague, a policy maker, or someone from the target population that you personally know.

Purposive Sampling

Purposive sampling is a nonprobability technique in which selection is based on the characteristics of the target population and the objectives of the study. This is particularly useful when you intend to select a small number of qualified participants for a study with a limited scope, which is often the case when using qualitative data collection methods. First, you set the qualifying criteria based on your assumptions about the target population. For example, if you assume that 20 percent of the target population is youth, then you need to enroll two youths out of each 10 participants. Second, you select only the kind of participants who are most relevant to the research objectives. For example, if you are assessing the quality of health care services, you need a sample of diverse individuals (patients, caregivers, physicians, nurses, etc.) with varied backgrounds, experiences, and roles. The goal is to select a sample that meets the variety of needs and assets of your study.

> *Example.* Kevin is a social worker who would like to understand the impact of a counseling program designed to improve the effectiveness of the welfare system on the lives of the recipients. He can only interview up to six households due to resource and logistical constraints. He decides to select his participants according to the following qualifying criteria: household size, parenting type (single parent, foster parents, etc.), and type of welfare program (housing assistance, MEDICAID, supplemental security income, etc.).

Reputational Sampling

Reputational sampling is a nonprobability technique that relies on finding the most knowledgeable participants in the context of their social network. You identify reputable key informants in your target population who may know more about the practice problem than the average participant. The objective here is to select a sample of participants who are most knowledgeable about a subject related to the entire target population.

Keep in mind that some participants will be reluctant to join a study or they may not show up for their appointments. This is a common problem, but you can address it in part by adopting an effective communication strategy. Individuals who are better informed and motivated are more likely to take part in the study and they can better help you achieve your research objectives. If they find your research relevant and beneficial, they are more likely to join and stay in the study. Research may not always directly benefit current participants; results are often used to enhance the quality of services for future clients/patients. However, many people choose to participate when they understand how their contributions are going to solve a problem and improve services.

One way of improving communication is to engage potential participants in the decision-making, hearing them out and addressing their points. This can significantly enhance the relevance of your research and the quality of communications about why the research is needed. Some individuals may want to join the study, but can't, because they are busy or have other obligations. Through effective communication, you can learn about those barriers (e.g., childcare, distance, timing) and make conscious efforts to address them by, for instance, scheduling the meeting(s) around their schedules, making childcare arrangements, or helping them with transportation. Lastly, you may decide to provide a small incentive (e.g., gift card or other type of reward) as a token of appreciation, which needs to be planned ahead of time and approved by management (and possibly by an ethical board) (see chapter 1). One important advantage of practitioner research, compared to other forms of research, is the close, everyday contact between the practitioner researcher and potential study participants. The practitioner researcher often already has a good working relationship with potential participants, making it more likely for them to agree to participate in research projects. The practitioner is also often aware of potential barriers to participation, making it easier to address these from the beginning.

4.4. Planning the Research Activities

After selecting data collection strategies and methods, it is time to list the research activities and create a work plan. The activities must include major logistical and supporting tasks that you need to do, such as enrollment, training, and communications. You also need to consider back-up plans and leave room for flexibility to adapt to unexpected events. Creating a work plan helps you organize the activities according to the desired implementation time frame, the status of each activity, and who is responsible for the activity. In a work plan, you list the activities in chronological order so those activities that are required to set the stage for other activities are accomplished first. In general, you may want to classify your activities based on their relevance to the plan as well as identify any necessary requirements and preconditions to carrying out the plan.

Describing Research Activities

Research activities are defined as actions that need to be carried out for successful implementation of a study, such as data collection, data analysis and conclusions, intervention development and testing, and documentation and presentation.

Data Collection

In practitioner research, your questions are important guides for identifying the type of needed data, collection methods, tools, and activities. It is often difficult to identify and organize all activities related to a specific data collection method, such as surveying clients/patients about the quality of services. Each method includes a series of activities that are either directly or indirectly related to data collection, such as recruitment, training, quality assurance, supervision and quality control, logistical considerations, and so on. Here we propose a way to facilitate the process of unpacking all activities associated with a data collection method. First, you need to list any methods that you have identified during previous activities. Second, use the following four questions for each data collection method to identify the activities.

1. *What is the question/sub-question associated with the data collection method?* Briefly describe the question and how it can be answered by data acquired from implementing the method. From the resulting data, describe any specific sub-questions that you wish to answer.

2. *What are the sources of the data?* List all sources of data that you intend to utilize. In general, there are two types of sources: preexisting material (written, visual, audio) and human participants. For each of the sources you need to determine (1) the target population and the sample population, and (2) the criteria for selecting relevant sources. In the case of preexisting material, this means identifying the larger body of material that you want to use and deciding whether you can use all the material, or if you need to use only certain pieces. In the case of human participants, this means identifying the group of people (or organizations) used and deciding if you will include everyone or if you need to select a smaller group for your study.

3. *How will you collect the data?* List all data collection activities and the instruments that you intend to use (see chapter 5 for more details). Consider important activities and sub-activities that need to be carried out. Think about a logical order for conducting the activities. For example, when conducting an interview, a logical order of activities could be developing an interview guide and testing it, interviewing the participants, writing the results or a report, and sharing the report with the study participants or your colleagues. In this example, the main activities are ordered, and you may decide to break some of the activities down into important sub-activities (e.g., interviewing the participants requires preparation, scheduling, training).

4. When will you carry out the research activities? You need to create a chronological timetable for the activities in the order that you want them to be implemented.

Other Final Stages

The next stages of practitioner research—analysis and conclusion, intervention development and testing, and documentation and presentation—each entail important activities that need to be planned the same way that you planned previous activities. List major activities relevant to each respective stage and indicate how and when you plan to carry them out. This will allow you to allocate sufficient time for analyzing data, drawing conclusions, and so on. For example, if you are planning activities related to designing an intervention, you must specify exactly when you intend to test the intervention. Each of these final steps will be fully discussed in the following chapters.

Exercise 3. Selecting and Describing Data Collection Methods (see page 118)

Creating a Work Plan

A work plan is a useful tool for organizing research activities and putting them in chronological order. It also helps visualize the scope of the work and determine if it's realistic and feasible to implement the activities during the specified time period. If not, you can further narrow down the research questions and revise the activities in the work plan. Research questions and activities are closely associated and amenable to changes based on what you learn on the ground and on feedback from others.

Example. A high school counselor wants to assess the life skills training needs of 15- to 18-year-old inner-city youth. He wants to use the results to design an intervention that would help the youth better navigate adverse life experiences outside the school environment. During his study's orientation and focusing stages, he observed a number of students in three after-school programs, studied relevant literature, and discussed the issues with parents and colleagues. After doing this, he came up with a long list of research activities that needed to be conducted. When he constructed the work plan, he realized that he had more activities planned than he could handle, and he wouldn't be able to answer his research question properly. This was mainly because the needs of the freshmen differ greatly from those of the seniors. Therefore, he decided to narrow down his research question to include only the freshmen, based on his observation that interventions when starting high school have an effect as the students become older. He made adjustments to the work plan to include only this group.

A detailed work plan of research activities could be used as a tool for communicating the research plan with others and soliciting their input. This can both enhance the quality of your research and generate more support for your research. Even for small studies, it is easy to overlook such details as a prescheduled event, sensitivity of certain topics, colleagues' possible reservations, and the lack of specific expertise.

A work plan can be constructed in different ways. One useful approach is a Gantt chart (table 4.1). This type of work plan looks like a calendar or a bar chart that illustrates the schedule of the activities. You can construct the chart using the table function in standard word processing programs (such as Word) or using database software (such as Excel).

Exercise 4. Planning Data Collection Methods (see page 118)

Table 4.1. Gantt chart

Category	Research activity	October 2022	November 2022
Data collection	Survey all clients		
Data collection	Focus groups with clients		
Analysis and conclusion	Generate summary of survey and focus group findings		
Documentation and presentation	Write up results and present results to clients and colleagues		

Identifying the Requirements for a Study

There are always basic requirements for each study. They include, but are not limited to, availability of resources, logistical and administrative support, necessary permissions, funding, and in-kind support. It would be wise to carefully identify the basic requirements for your research and to make sure that they are in place before implementing your project. This can save you time and effort. Share your ideas and plans with colleagues and management so you can better understand everything you need, take care of any deficiencies, and avoid stagnation at a later stage due to time or resource constraints.

The following questions can help you identify the requirements of your research:

How much time do you and your colleagues need to spend on the research project?

How do you log the time spent on research (as working hours or personal time)?

What type of instruments, tools, and materials need to be purchased? How much do they cost? Who is paying for them?

Where will the research activities take place? Are all needed locations available?

What is the impact of the research on the workflow of the organization?

How much will the research cost? What kind of funding or in-kind support is available to you?

What kind of approval (e.g., administrative, ethical) do you need for the project, and for what parts?

Do you have permission to utilize the organization's resources and communication tools to reach out to colleagues, clients/patients, and other stakeholders?

What kinds of technical and administrative support do you have?

Who are your most important contact persons when you need help?

4.5. The Research Plan

A research plan is a summary of the activities that you have done during the orientation, focusing, and planning stages of the Practitioner Research Method. It is an overview of the problem analysis and all planned elements of the practitioner research study, justifications for selected data collections methods, a statement of how the study's findings will be applied, and the study's potential benefits. The practice problem and the research objectives determine the scope of your research plan.

Example 1. Sandy is a junior counselor who works in a residential at-risk youth program, serving adolescents struggling with emotional and behavioral issues. She has difficulty convincing the young residents to take more responsibility for household chores and to work as a team. Many of the residents don't follow the agreement regarding their responsibilities, telling her that they have never done any chores in their lives. She decides to conduct a descriptive study to explore various ways of fostering interest among the residents and promoting follow-through with the basic rules of the facility. First, she reviews relevant literature on this topic to expand her knowledge. Then, she interviews a few of her senior colleagues. As a result, Sandy comes up with promising tips and ideas that she compiles into a set of guidelines. The guidelines are very well-received during a team meeting and adopted as materials that will be used for training other counselors.

In this example, Sandy's research has a limited scope and a succinct research plan is enough. Sandy is conducting her research to enhance her own professional competency, and she used the research plan as a tool to achieve that.

Example 2. Malcolm conducts research in the final year of his public health program. He is doing an internship as a health educator at a Head Start program in El Paso. He wants to design a health education program for parents that focuses on healthy diet and active lifestyles. Most staff find his idea beneficial and timely. A few colleagues, however, express concern over the lack of required expertise in serving families from cultural minority backgrounds. Malcolm drafts a research plan that aims at improving the parents' dietary behaviors and level of physical activity after participating in a lifestyle education program. He works with a few families from various cultural backgrounds for six months to better understand their needs and develop the curriculum. The results help him design a coaching program. He tests his approach and makes adaptations to the program based on input from experts and the families involved in the study. He asks the parents to keep a journal and document the positive and negative aspects of the coaching program. At the end of the project, Malcolm studies the impact of the intervention on each family. He summarizes his findings in a report and gives a presentation about his new coaching program to the staff.

This second example is about a more substantive research project than the previous one, with a wider scope. Malcolm needed a detailed research plan because he had to explore the subject, describe his research objectives, design a new method, and test the model on a few eligible families. Furthermore, as an intern, Malcolm needed to fulfil the academic expectations of his school and do something relevant to the needs of the Head Start program.

Elements of a Research Plan

The outline of a research plan usually includes the following sections or elements:
1. Introduction
2. Practice problem
3. Research strategy

These sections are interrelated and based on the stages of practitioner research. Therefore, changes in any one section of the plan usually lead to changes in other sections.

For example, as you progress and gain new insights, you might want to revise one of your research activities. This means that you also need to review and revise the corresponding research question, add more relevant literature, and revise the work plan.

Outline of a Research Plan

1. Introduction
    a. Significance

    Clearly indicate the significance of your research. What was the reason for conducting this research? Was it self-initiated or were you asked to conduct the research? If asked, who made the request and why? What is your motivation for doing this research? Who will benefit from the results, and how?

    b. Setting

    Broadly define the research setting. Describe specific characteristics of the setting that are relevant to your research, such as: the nature, structure, and size of the organization; the clients/patients, and other beneficiaries; other stakeholders and collaborators; and, a description of the outside community.

    c. The research team

    Briefly introduce your fellow researchers, the person or the department that requested the research, and the organization's resources and capacity for conducting research.

    d. Alignment with internal policies and procedures

    Explain how your research is aligned with the organization's policies and, when applicable, any past research. Describe your plan for minimizing possible interruptions to organizational procedures and workflow. Discuss the benefits of the research, and its impact on the growth and development of the organization and the quality of services.

2. Practice Problem
    a. Description of the practice problem

    Describe the practice problem based on the 6W+H method in chapter 2.

    b. Literature review

    Provide an overview of your findings related to the key aspects of the practice problem, any themes and sub-themes, and their interrelationships. Describe how the information presented in the literature relates to your practice problem. Always refer to your sources and cite them properly. Discuss how the literature review informs the practice problem. Discuss any contributing factors, possible solutions, key themes and sub-themes, and relationships between various components related to your topic.

c. Research objective

Clearly explain what you aim to accomplish through your research and its potential benefits to the organization and to you personally.

d. Research question

Clearly articulate the main questions and possible sub-questions of your research and define any significant concepts.

3. Research Strategy

a. Research activities

In this section, you are supposed to report your research activities, their relevance to the research questions, your data sources, and the order of the activities in a work plan format. Start with describing your data collection methods, using the following questions to help you more thoroughly report the necessary components of your data collection activities:

- What are the associations between your questions, sub-questions, and selected data collection methods?
- Which sources of data do you use in the research?
- Through what research activities are you planning to collect data?
- What is the timeline of the research activities?

Likewise, describe your planned activities and their timelines related to analysis and conclusions, intervention design and testing (when applicable), and documentation and presentation.

b. Work plan

Put the research activities in a work plan using a Gantt chart or another planning format of your choosing, such as a timeline chart or a flowchart.

c. Requirements

Explain the requirements for the successful implementation of your research activities. Describe the nature of the requirements and why they are necessary. Commonly these include, but are not limited to, availability of resources, logistical and administrative support, necessary permissions, funding, other in-kind support, and any extra time and/or financial resources you need to achieve the desired research results.

Evaluate the Research Plan

Evaluation of your research plan is a very important step that could significantly improve the quality of your work. Furthermore, evaluation is often a requirement of grant funding, internships, or course assignments. Organizations may set their own evaluation criteria. To conduct a self-assessment of your plan, we recommend the following criteria:

Are all sections or elements of the research plan clearly described?

Do the contents of the sections or elements follow a coherent and logical argument?

Will you be able to answer the research questions by completing the activities?

Is the work plan realistic and feasible?

Have you ensured sufficient triangulation?

Do you maintain ethical boundaries and comply with privacy and data use laws?

Do you expect the research activities to provide you and/or others with new insights?

Are the research activities clearly described in a way that other parties can fully understand them?

Are communications and self-reflection activities part of the plan? Are they scheduled appropriately?

Have stakeholders in the organization read your research plan? Do they support your plan?

Does the research plan also have

- a cover page with essential information (e.g., title of the project, researchers' names and contact information);
- a table of contents;
- page numbers;
- a list of references and sources (see appendix);
- the correct format; and
- no editorial and grammatical errors?

Exercise 5. Drafting a Work Plan (see page 118)

Exercise 6. Evaluating a Research Plan (see page 119)

4.6. Summary

Data collection methods are selected according to their expected capacity to help you find answers to your research questions. It is advised to employ as many feasible methods as possible so you can triangulate the results and reach more valid and reliable conclusions. Your questions and sub-questions reflect whether you want to either describe, define, compare, evaluate, or explain, which in turn determines the type of data that you will need to collect.

In this chapter we described and compared types of data collection, which include document analysis, systematic observation (of people and situations), interviewing, surveying, testing, alternative methods, and site visits. Data collection can be qualitative or quantitative in nature, or a combination of both (*mixed methods*) can be used in one study.

In practitioner research you collect most data from people (respondents/participants), but you may also use preexisting material (textual, visual, audio). It is not always feasible to include your entire target population. Therefore, you often need to draw a representative sample based on random, probability, or nonprobability sampling techniques.

Creating a work plan for the planned research activities was discussed using a Gantt chart. Furthermore, the importance of identifying the requirements for your project was discussed, along with ideas for ensuring that they are in place so research results can be achieved according to the plan.

The research plan summarizes the activities conducted during the orientation, focusing and planning stages of practitioner research, and these components were outlined in the last section of this chapter. Your plan is a foundation for the implementation of your research, and it should entail what you wish to research, how you plan to carry out the research, and how much time you think you will need. A research plan comprises (a) an introduction, (b) a practice problem, and (c) a research strategy. It is highly recommended to discuss your research plan with other colleagues and stakeholders so you can both improve it, based on their feedback, and generate more support. You can also assess your research plan yourself by checking it against the set of self-assessment evaluation criteria provided.

EXERCISES

Exercise 1. Evaluating Selected Data Collection Method(s)

Discuss the strengths and weaknesses of the following set of data collection methods with one of your colleagues.

> Fred is a nurse working in a community hospital in New Orleans. He has drafted the following research questions:
>
> How much do nurses know about the hospital's patient safety policy?
>
> How well do they implement it in their daily practices?
>
> Fred's first step is to ask all nurses in the hospital to respond to a questionnaire to find out how much they are aware of and know about the hospital's patient safety policy. Then, he invites four nurses from one department to a group discussion to explore how well the policy is implemented. Fred has developed the questionnaire and the interview guides based on the patient safety policy document. He has neither shared nor discussed his questionnaire or interview guide with his colleagues or supervisor.

Exercise 2. Generating a Client/Patient Summary Report

A client/patient summary report is a document that provides a comprehensive overview of a client/patient's care. The report is generated from data collected through various methods, and the client/patient is the primary source. Data is mainly collected through client/patient observation, client/patient interviews (individually or in a group session), and client/patient records (files, reports, logs).

Identify three fictional clients/patients, and through discussion with colleagues give each of them a unique problem and a history of care. Each of you will separately prepare a short bio for each patient using information that you supposedly have gained from records review, observation, and formal and informal interviews. After finishing the bios, compile yours into a summary report. Each of your colleagues will do the same for the bios they have written.

Compare your individually compiled bios and summary reports to identify commonalities and differences. Discuss the differences.

Exercise 3. Selecting and Describing Data Collection Methods

This is a group exercise that needs to be performed with other teammates. Prior to the meeting, each member drafts a research question relevant to the organization. At the meeting, members give brief presentations to share the questions and their significance. After the presentations, members are given a few minutes to individually list research activities relevant to each suggested question. Then they share their list with the group. At the end, each participant chooses the three most appropriate and effective research activities for each research question and discusses them with the rest of the group.

Exercise 4. Planning Data Collection Methods

Rasheed and Peter are interested in exploring the cultural competency of case managers and community health workers (CHWs) in a mental health clinic in Austin, Texas. Rasheed wants to start by surveying a large group of case managers and CHWs, followed by a few individual in-depth interviews with supervisors. Peter, on the other hand, prefers the exact opposite approach. He suggests starting with a few individual interviews with supervisors followed by a group discussion with the case managers and CHWs. He believes that his approach can better clarify the issues and the need for conducting a survey.

What is your opinion of these suggested data collection activities? Spend a little time to clarify your position and discuss your reasons with one of your colleagues. Listen to your colleague's comments and try to build consensus on a reasonable approach for the study.

Exercise 5. Drafting a Work Plan

There is an ongoing conflict between the staff and visitors of a nursing home. The problem analysis shows that visitors often file complaints about the attitude and behaviors of the staff after asking them questions. The visitors feel that the staff do not take their questions seriously and are not helpful. The staff often argue that they are very busy and cannot spend much time answering every question.

Draft an appropriate research question for the above scenario with the objective of improving the relationship between visitors and the staff. Choose your data collection methods and write down a few research activities that can help answer the question. Create a realistic work plan for the research activities.

If you are doing this exercise as a team, compare different work plans constructed by each member and discuss the similarity and differences between the suggested research activities.

Exercise 6. Evaluating a Research Plan

Follow the self-assessment evaluation criteria to assess one or more research plans. You can use research plans from previous studies, your own research plan, or research plans developed by colleagues.

REFERENCES

Bold, C. (2012). *Using narrative in research*. Sage.

Delnooz, P. (2010). *Creatieve actie methodologie* [Creative action methodology]. Boom Lemma.

Geenen, M. (2017). *Reflecteren: Leren van je ervaringen als sociale professional* [Reflection: Learning from your experiences as a social professional]. Bussum: Coutinho.

Goodman, L. A. (1961). Snowball sampling. *Annals of Mathematical Statistics, 32*(1), 148–170. https://doi.org/10.1214/aoms/1177705148

Lorenz, L. S., & Kolb, B. (2009). Involving the public through participatory visual research methods. *Health Expectations, 12*(3), 262–274. https://doi.org/10.1111/j.1369-7625 .2009.00560.x

Packard, J. (2008). "I'm gonna show you what it's really like out here": The power and limitation of participatory visual methods. *Visual Studies, 23*(1), 63–77. https://doi.org/10.1080 /14725860801908544

Ledwith, M., & Springett, J. (2010). *Participatory practice: Community-based action for transformative change*. Policy Press.

Van Biene, M., Kohlmann, J., Heessels, M., Bobbink, E., Degen-Nijeboer, H., Geurts, E., Pelzer, M., & Woudenberg, J. (2012). *Narratief! Wablief? Ieder zijn eigen verhaal* [Narratives! What do you mean? Everyone his or her own story]. Hogeschool van Arnhem en Nijmegen.

Von Unger, H. (2013). *Partizipative Forschung: Einführung in die Forschungspraxis* [Participatory research: An introduction to research practice]. Springer VS.

5

Data Collection

When your research plan is finalized, it basically means that you have identified and planned all necessary activities to answer the research question. This chapter focuses on the data collection component of the research plan and provides tools and activities that can be used in professional practice settings (figure 5.1). Data collection instruments are discussed first, followed by further exploration of the main types of data collection used in practitioner research: document analysis, systematic observation, interviewing, surveying, testing, alternative methods, and site visits. A summary of the chapter and relevant exercises are provided at the end.

5.1. Data Collection Instruments

Data collection in practitioner research is a means to an end: to learn more about a practice problem that we don't fully understand. The practice problem informs the research question that is expected to be answered through accurate and consistent data

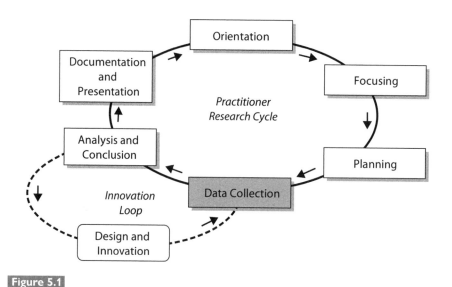

Figure 5.1

Key component of practitioner research: Data Collection

collected via suitable instruments and methods. Using reliable and tested tools—such as observation charts, a log or a journal, a review outline, interview guides, validated tests, or questionnaires—will help you to collect accurate data. Many useful and standardized instruments are readily available and many of them may have already become part of an organization's standard operating procedures (clinical charts, progress notes, evaluation forms, patient satisfaction questionnaires, etc.).

If you are conducting research on a new subject and you cannot find a suitable instrument to use, you can adapt an existing instrument or develop a new tool.

Quantitative Instruments

In quantitative instruments, the responses or options are predefined, and the responses can be numerical data or data that can be converted into numbers. These types of questions consist of numerical questions and closed questions, with three specific types of closed questions: single-choice, multiple-response, and scaled (i.e., choosing one option from a range of ordered options). For the scaled options, which are also referred to as Likert scales, respondents are urged to report the intensity of their feelings or of the situation by choosing from a range, for instance, "very low to very high" or "strongly disagree to strongly agree." Such ranges can have an odd number of options (three, five, seven, or nine) with the middle item being a neutral response (e.g., "neither agree nor disagree").

The disadvantage of having a neutral category is that the participant in your study may choose that option if they are unsure how to respond. By having an even number of options, the participant is forced to choose a response that points in one direction or the other. The disadvantage to an even number of options is that participants who truly have a neutral position do not find an answer corresponding to how they feel. You can test which number of options is best by doing a pilot test (more on those later). In any case, it is recommended to always include an additional item to scaled options so that participants who are not certain of their answer will find an appropriate response (e.g., "not applicable" or "not sure").

Qualitative Instruments

Qualitative questions are open-ended, not limited to a set of predetermined options. The items of the qualitative instruments for document analysis, systematic observations, and surveys or interviews are different in nature but they all lead to data in the form of words, phrases, passages, or even documents. Qualitative data are usually processed and analyzed using codes and themes but can sometimes be quantified by counting instances of codes and themes if needed.

Later in this chapter you will learn how to design different types of quantitative and qualitative instruments for document analysis, systematic observation, and interviews, surveys, or tests. Examples of instruments using various focal points, areas of observation, and questions will be provided along with their resulting information and analytical methods. Therefore, by the end of this chapter, you will be ready to learn how to analyze your data, which is the focus of chapter 6.

Developing an Instrument for Data Collection

To design a data collection instrument from scratch, follow these steps:

1. Identify a research question.

2. Select an appropriate data collection method, which can be document analysis, systematic observation, interviewing, surveying, or testing.

3. List key aspects and sub-themes that you have identified through the literature review.

4. The sub-themes are further broken down (*operationalized*) into instrument items: focal points (in document analysis), areas of observation (in systematic observation) and/or questions (in interviews and surveys). Such items can inform the design of quantitative or qualitative instruments leading to numerical data or textual data.

Example. Donna is a nurse working in a Planned Parenthood health care center in Los Angeles. She is in charge of a program that provides reproductive health care services to adolescents and young adults. Her research question is "What are the clients' perceptions of the family planning counseling session they attended?" To answer the question, she intends to interview a few clients immediately after the counseling session, so she needs an interview guide.

Donna has not found a suitable interview guide on this topic and decides to create her own. Through her literature review, she identified the following key aspects (and sub-themes): satisfaction (interaction with the counselor, the quality of the information, the venue), usefulness (new knowledge, new ideas, intention to change), concerns (areas not covered, nonrelevant subjects, poor quality), and suggestions. She writes down the key aspects and sub-themes in an outline format (i.e., lists the sub-themes under their respective key aspects). Lastly, she lists the instrument components (e.g., counselor's attitude, listening, attention, knowledge) under the relevant sub-themes.

A step-by-step plan for developing various types of data collection instruments is described here and illustrated in table 5.1. And an example of creating an observation chart based on the first six steps of this instrument development guide is provided in table 5.2. Like previous stages, the process starts with the definition of the practice problem.

Developing Data Collection Instruments: A Step-by-Step Guide

1. Create a table with four columns.

2. In column one, write down the purpose of the instrument.

3. In column two, list the key aspects related to the purpose. Your problem analysis and the respective research question are primary sources for identifying the key aspects.

4. In column three, note any sub-themes related to the data collection's key aspects.

5. In column four, state each sub-theme in the format for how you will use it in the instrument as a focal point for document analysis, an area of observation, and/or an interview or survey question. The resulting statement can be a phrase, a sentence, or a question.

6. Review all the items (focal points, areas of observation, and/or questions) and select those that are most relevant to the purpose, the key aspects, and the sub-themes.

7. Create your desired instrument (e.g., comparison chart, observation checklist, interview guide, questionnaire), using selected items from the fourth column. Try to match your writing to the literacy level and language of your participants. Put the questions in a logical order and clarify any ambiguities or difficult terms.

8. Conduct a pilot test (also called a pre-test) whenever possible to assess the usefulness (validity) of the instrument and enhance its accuracy (reliability). You can test your instrument with documents you want to include in your study (in the case of a document analysis), by trying it out in an appropriate place (in the case of observations), or by administering it to potential participants (in the case of interviews, surveys, or tests). The pilot test usually reveals problems with the instrument (e.g., certain topics are missing, certain questions are not understandable, or participants are unclear on instructions).

Table 5.1. Template for creating a research instrument

Purpose of the data collection instrument	Key aspects	Sub-themes	Instrument items (focal points for document analysis, areas of observation, interview/survey/test questions)
Purpose 1	Key aspect 1	Sub-theme 1.1	
		Sub-theme 1.2	
	Key aspect 2	Sub-theme 2.1	
		Sub-theme 2.2	
		Sub-theme 2.3	

Table 5.2. An observation chart in progress

Purpose of the observation	Key aspects	Sub-themes	Observational points
To observe the quality of patient-provider interactions in a prenatal care unit.	Issues discussed	Lifestyle changes	The provider clearly explains healthy lifestyle behaviors during the pregnancy related to diet, exercise, stress, and work.
		Required tests and medications	The provider clearly communicates all the tests and medical interventions during the prenatal visits.
		Safe pregnancy	The provider explains all danger signs and symptoms, such as bleeding, infection, high blood pressure, etc.
			The provider gives tips on how to identify danger signs and symptoms and on when to seek help.
	The quality of the interaction	Reflective listening	The provider allows the client to freely discuss her questions and then the provider paraphrases some of the key points to make sure that she understands the questions.
		Rapport	The conversations are conducted in a relaxed and friendly environment where the client and the provider seem to be at ease and understand each other.

Important Instrument Development Tips

Always remember to avoid collecting irrelevant and/or unnecessary data. The following example illustrates how to collect useful information:

Example. Counselors working with a psychologist to run a support group at a juvenile detention center have reported conflicts between group members. The counselor asks the attending psychologist to exclude a few specific members from the group. The psychologist decides to independently investigate the problem. She asks each member of the group to answer the following two questions: "Who do you spend most of your time with?" and "Who would you rather not hang out with?" She draws a table showing how often each member is mentioned by peers and in which context. This approach helps her to understand if the problem is an isolated event resulting from one or two individuals or a systemic phenomenon.

Also keep in mind that an instrument must be intentionally designed to facilitate data analysis. Your data collection method must be aligned with your selected analytical approach, otherwise you could run into serious problems.

Example. You want to learn more about your case managers' perceptions of their assigned workloads. To achieve this objective, you conduct two different types of surveys. You ask half of the case managers if they are able to complete their assignments within the expected time frame. The other half you ask how much time they usually have outside of work to spend with friends and family.

In this example, the separate questions asked of the two halves of the group are aligned. However, although the themes are related, the resulting data are not easily comparable.

Even if the questions used for two groups are the same, if the format of the response sets differ, it will be quite difficult to compare the results.

Example. Nurses who work in the surgery department are asked question X, while pediatric nurses are asked question Y.

Question X: My workload is high.

    Completely agree   1   2   3   4   5   Completely disagree

Question Y: My workload is high.

- o Always
- o Sometimes
- o Rarely

In this case, you will find it difficult during the data analysis stage of research to compare the answers from these two groups mainly because, in reality, you have asked two different questions.

The following sections provide a few examples of useful instruments for document analysis, systematic observation, interviewing, surveying, testing, and site visits. Through the examples, you will learn how to draft and finalize quantitative and qualitative focal points, areas of observation, and/or questions.

5.2. Document Analysis

The process of document analysis includes reviewing and evaluating public, internal, and other textual sources (see appendix). In this section, we explain how to design an instrument for analyzing and reviewing documents.

Example. A survey shows that nurses of a geriatric clinic feel they are not adequately equipped to deal with elderly patients suffering from basophobia (fear of falling). The team wants to design an instrument for analyzing the scientific literature and clinic documents based on the following question: "How can nurses more effectively identify and address basophobia among elderly patients?"

A related sub-question to the above example is: "What are the characteristics, causes, signs, and symptoms of basophobia in patients over 65 years of age?" After a document analysis, the nurses intend to conduct a few interviews with elderly patients and observe their daily activities. The sequence of these activities is carefully considered. Information gained through document analysis provides insight into basophobia among the elderly, which can then be used as a starting point for conducting the interviews and the observation.

Besides published literature, document analysis instruments can be used for other sources of data (service statistics, evaluation reports, meeting notes, patient progress notes, etc.). For example, a social worker who works at a youth development center can review the center's online discussion board and emails to identify clients' frequently asked questions.

Selecting a Document Analysis Approach

Various sources can be used to answer a sub-question that requires document analysis. To start, a set of *inclusion and exclusion criteria* can clarify what sources you want or do not want to use (table 5.3). They also enable you to specify why you do or do not include certain sources.

To make your work replicable by others, you must document important details about the approach you used (e.g., your search strategy) for finding your sources. For example, if you are interested in finding laws and regulations on a specific topic, you may want to start by analyzing the policy documents of relevant agencies.

When you search any databases or search engines, documenting the queries and the number of hits you get for each search can be useful (table 5.4). This will help others understand the way that you have broadened or narrowed the scope of the search based on the results. In most search engines, you can use advanced options that allow for more precise searches, such as including, combining, or excluding certain terms or keywords.

Table 5.3. Example of inclusion and exclusion criteria for sources related to a hypothetical research project	
Inclusion criteria	Exclusion criteria
The source is:	The source:
about inpatient services	is about minors (people less than 18 years old)
on quality of life	
available in full text	was published before 2005

Table 5.4. Varying queries and documenting the number of hits they each have during a document search	
Query	Number of hits
Nurses	119,098
Nurses AND empathy	1,992
Nurses AND empathy AND infant	313
Nurses AND empathy AND infant NOT birth	101

For internal documents, you often need creative strategies different than those used when searching the scientific literature. The strategy you use will largely depend on how documents are stored and catalogued.

Follow the instructions in the appendix to assess the reliability and usefulness of the sources that you find.

Developing a Document Analysis Instrument

Promising sources need to be analyzed in depth. A *comparison chart* is a useful tool for examining the strengths, weaknesses, and overall usefulness of the sources for inclusion. For example, the comparison chart in table 5.5 was used to examine a training manual on self-reliance among 16- to 21-year-old youths diagnosed with Autism Spectrum Disorder (ASD). It contains open-ended (qualitative) focal points and is only a portion of a larger instrument. Compare this to the chart used by a nurse to study the frequency and type of documented nursing errors in 2019 (table 5.6). She used the chart to calculate the frequency of the incidents, the types of errors, and actions taken following each incident (quantitative focal points).

The focal points used in any comparison chart can be quantitative or qualitative statements or questions.

Table 5.5. Self-reliance comparison chart using open-ended focal points

Sub-question: What topics are discussed in the manual?	Description
1 How does the source describe social interactions?	
2 What information is provided on teaching planning and organizational skills?	
3 How does the source address the issue of achieving a realistic vision for future treatments?	

Table 5.6. Nursing errors comparison chart capturing quantitative focal points

Sub-question: How many cases of nursing errors have been reported in 2019 (per incident category)?	Frequency
1 Administration of wrong medications	
2 Provision of incorrect foods, diet, or nutrition education	
3 Accidental falls and injuries on the part of patients	
4 Miscommunication-related incidents	
5 Conducting inappropriate examinations	
6 Conducting incorrect interventions	

Numerical Focal Point: Examples

What percentage of the content is about stereotyping and discrimination?

How many discussed topics are listed in the meeting notes?

Closed-Option Focal Point: Examples

Single-option focal point

The document is written in

- ○ English
- ○ Spanish
- ○ Other languages

Multiple-option focal point

What topics have been listed in the staff satisfaction questionnaire? (please check all that apply)

- ☐ Workload
- ☐ Role and responsibility
- ☐ Autonomy
- ☐ Teamwork
- ☐ Multiplicity of duties
- ☐ Transparency
- ☐ Trust
- ☐ Job security

Scaled Focal Point: Example

The instructions were clear as to how friends and relatives are kept informed of your well-being.

Completely agree   1   2   3   4   5   Completely disagree

Open-Ended Focal Point: Examples

What is the position of the author on using electronic devices in informal care?

What strategies are suggested in the source for meeting the needs of men and women during a counseling session?

The focal points help identify and mark useful answers, phrases, or text fragments while performing document analysis. In section 5.1, a step-by-step plan for selecting the focal points was described. Use a proper citation format to refer to and list the original sources in your notes during the data collection process (see appendix). Structured comparison charts can significantly improve the quality of the data collection process and provide a useful framework for analyzing the data.

5.3. Systematic Observation

In practitioner research, systematic observation means purposefully viewing and analyzing situations or events that occur during professional practice. Some types of research questions can be more effectively answered through systematic observation of certain events, especially when guided by suitable tools. Through observation, you can learn more deeply about what really happens in professional practice on a daily basis.

Decisions around "who makes the observations," "what is observed," and "how to do it" are answered according to the objective of the observation and the respective research question and sub-questions. The subjects of the observation are often the behavior of providers and their patients/clients in health care and social work settings.

Example. Linda is a freshman majoring in physical therapy who is doing an internship in a health care center. One of her assignments is to attend and observe her supervisor's treatment sessions. Linda writes down important details of what she observes about the treatment and her supervisor's interactions with the patients.

Linda's free or unstructured observation technique is a common practice. She doesn't have a specific objective in mind and writes down every detail that seems important to her. Sometimes in exploratory studies, it's beneficial to enter an arena and start observing without any set preconceptions. However, it would save time and be wiser, in most situations, to conduct observations with a specific objective in mind. A clear definition of the objective in the example of Linda, for instance, could shift attention toward the supervisor's behavior, the interaction between the supervisor and the patients, or the patient responses to and compliance with the treatment. The objective could be stated as "How does the supervisor manage his time?" or "How much feedback does the supervisor provide to the patients?" or "What is the level of compliance to the treatment among the patients?"

Identify the behaviors you intend to observe prior to the session (see section 5.1). For instance, if you are interested in learning team leader techniques for facilitating groups in a drug recovery center, your focus should be on their skills and facilitation activities. Or, if you are interested in assessing how much the health care staff follow the safety and sanitation protocol, you would need to focus on actions related to safe practices and personal hygiene. Such observation activities can reinforce information found in the scientific literature and internal documents. For instance, in the latter case, you may be able to find detailed information about facilitation techniques and policy documents on safety and sanitation.

Prior to observation, you must specify where the observation can take place. For example, team leader facilitation techniques can be observed during a support group meeting that is facilitated by a team leader, during a performance review session where a team leader and their supervisors meet, or in a training session where the team leaders role-play.

Plan your observation method only after having a clear objective statement, identifying the behaviors to be observed, and specifying the situations where the behaviors can be observed.

Selecting the Observation Approach

Systematic observations can be performed in various ways, which are determined by the specific situation, possible limitations, and the type and scope of the research question and sub-questions (Flick, 2014; Stokking, 2000):

Single vs. multiple observations

Participant vs. nonparticipant observation

Direct vs. indirect observation

Less-structured vs. structured observation

These approaches are not exclusive and can overlap. Furthermore, Flick (2014) introduces the following additions to the list:

Open vs. hidden observation

Observation in natural settings vs. controlled environments (field vs. lab)

Third party observation vs. self-observation

In total, these approaches lend themselves to numerous combinations and options, so you can identify the approach that is most relevant for your research. For example, you can use a single observation approach that is structured, direct, participatory, and conducted in a natural setting.

Single vs. Multiple Observations

Depending on your objective, sometimes you may be able to acquire enough data by performing a single observation, or maybe the event is a unique one (e.g., observing a special occasion, such as a student graduation ceremony). However, you may need multiple observations over a longer period of time to fully understand a situation and answer your research question. Repeated observations of the same variables over long periods of time is called *longitudinal observation,* which is often used when you want to track the effects of an intervention.

> *Example.* A geriatric psychiatry team wants to assess the effectiveness of their novel training called "Dealing with Fear." They perform two observations of the elderly participants, one before and one after the training session.

Repeated observations can be regarded as a more robust approach compared to a single observation as it often leads to a more accurate understanding of the variations that exist in real-life situations.

Example. A student intern who is majoring in health education performs a single observation of the residents of an assisted living facility while engaged in recreational activities. Only three residents are present on that Friday afternoon. He concludes that the residents do not sufficiently make use of the recreational activities and programs.

Obviously, a single observation on one Friday afternoon cannot sufficiently provide you with the full picture. There is a chance that more residents may engage in the activities on other days and at other times. It is also possible that other concurrent activities might have been scheduled on that specific Friday afternoon.

In contrast, the following example describes a case where multiple observations have been performed:

Example. Two medical students in a community hospital are asked to perform multiple observations of one individual patient in recovery. The objective is to chart the patient's well-being and performance during the assigned activities. First, each student performs the observation independently and then they share their notes. Both students use the same tool and at the end of each observation they discuss their consolidated results with the attending physician. The students perform multiple observations of the same patient on different days and during various activities over a three-week period.

Participant vs. Nonparticipant Observation

Participant observation applies to situations where the researcher chooses to be an active participant in the observed process. In *nonparticipant observation*, the researcher observes from the outside. Participant observation is often a more realistic choice for health care and social work settings where there are more things to do than to merely observe.

In a way, a participant observation can be regarded as half observation and half interview, which allows for a more elaborate examination of the professional practice. This form of observation has been commonly used by ethnographers in their efforts to map a community's assets from an insider's perspective. Through participant observation, you can develop a more realistic view of community structures and/or relationships by experiencing them firsthand. Where necessary, you can ask for clarification or feedback during the observation.

The problem with participant observation is that in some situations your participation may change the nature of the services; you may also lack awareness of certain aspects of what is going on because you are in the midst of the activity. The results will be valid only in situations where the observed practices are part of the routine activities, your interactions won't influence the care dynamic, and you are careful to reflect on how being part of the activity affects what you observe. During participant observation, you often perform more than one activity simultaneously, such as "observing and providing care," "observing and participating in a discussion," or "observing and counseling." It is important to carefully plan the logistical details prior to the observation, such as how you will document the observations and how you will keep records.

In nonparticipant observation, you are not an active part of the observed situation. Rather, the research is performed at a distance so that the observation does not change the participants' normal behavior.

> *Example.* You intend to learn about an autistic child's attention span and capacity. Instead of engaging with the child or playing a game while observing her and making notes about the frequency and duration of her attention (participant approach), using a nonparticipant approach, you don't have any active role and merely observe the child's interaction with the environment and other children from a distance, or maybe from another room through a one-way mirror.

Either way, you are ethically obliged to explain the objective of your intended participant or nonparticipant observations and provide written information and consent forms beforehand.

Direct vs. Indirect Observation

Direct observation is about watching an event live and firsthand with all senses involved, which is important for understanding the full picture by noting details such as sounds, smells, or body language. Through direct observation, you can actively choose what to observe and where to pay more attention.

> *Example.* A speech therapist wants to learn how the oral/aural and lip-reading methods are implemented at a center for deaf and hard-of-hearing education by observing a few sessions conducted by two experienced colleagues. During the sessions, she sits in the back of the room and observes attentively.

By definition, when you directly observe an event you only have the one chance to see what takes place. Therefore, you must clearly and thoroughly document your observations without any delays. Another approach, joint observation, can be logistically difficult since both observers need to be present at the same time and their presence may more significantly affect the behavior of the participants. On the other hand, one observer may not be able to pay attention and document all important details when several participants interact at the same time.

In *indirect observation,* the researcher usually video or audio records the session for later viewing of the event. This could be used as a stand-alone approach or mixed with direct observation to complement the results and enable further viewing and examination.

> *Example.* Dana is a social worker assigned to help a couple provide support to their foster child who suffers from post-traumatic stress disorder. He suggests that they record a video of their child during select daily indoor and outdoor activities. They review the video and use it to develop a therapy plan. In addition, he asks for permission to record their counseling session and show both videos to his colleagues. He and his colleagues observe the video, share their thoughts, and reach a conclusion.

Indirect observation has the following advantages:

- Lower odds of interfering with the natural dynamics of the event by not being visibly present.
- Unlimited viewing of / listening to recorded materials is possible, if needed.
- The possibility of more than one individual observing or performing joint observations followed by validating the findings through intersubjectivity and triangulation.
- Allowing for observing at a later time while actively participating in the event (participant observation).

Indirect observation has some notable disadvantages, too, mostly related to logistical aspects and ethical dilemmas of audio and video recording. If confidentiality or topic sensitivity preclude recording, you may miss valuable data. For example, important details could be overlooked, such as hard-to-capture body language clues, muted sounds, scents, or simultaneous nearby events.

Less-Structured vs. Structured Observation

Professional practice events can be observed in ways that are less structured or fully structured. *Less-structured observations* are not restricted by any particular focus, so they allow for a more diverse collection of observations. The objective of less-structured observations is usually exploratory in nature and more flexible.

Example. Shannon is a nurse practitioner who works at a hospital with an explicit core value of providing patient-centered care. But the definition of "patient-centered care" has not been clearly described. Shannon suggests the following question for research on this issue: What would be a clear definition of patient-centered care and its main characteristics? To answer the question, she invites four colleagues to observe each other while they are engaged in patient care. Their job is to write down observable aspects of the services that in their opinion are integral parts of patient-centered care. Based on the observation reports, Shannon drafts a description of how patient-centered care is interpreted.

In *structured observation*, you often use highly defined instruments that explicitly indicate specific aspects of the observed behavior. Here you must describe every focal point as concretely as possible to make sure that the focus of the observation is clear throughout the process. Your colleagues or fellow students all need to focus on the same aspects or behaviors during joint observations. In structured observations, data are often recorded using checklists, tally marks, or numbers.

Hidden Observation

Participants of a hidden observation are not aware of when and how they are observed. For ethical reasons, this form of observation is less common, as the persons being observed have not consented to participating in your study. The advantage of hidden observations is that people's behavior is not influenced by knowing they are being observed. Generally, hidden observations are carried out in public places, such as shopping malls, supermarkets, and parks, because making observations in such places usually does not require people's consent, nor does it impinge on other ethical considerations.

Observation in Natural Settings vs. Controlled Environments (Field vs. Lab)

Practitioner research studies are mostly conducted in natural, uncontrolled settings, which means that the events occur even if you don't observe them. In some other situations, settings can be intentionally created for social experiments or role-plays in order to answer specific questions that require controlled environments.

> *Example.* A social work professional is trying to learn how local residents react to certain everyday stressors in their neighborhood. He invites a group of residents to a meeting and asks them to engage in role-plays according to a few given scenarios. Then he performs a direct nonparticipant observation on how they act, based on those fictional cases.

Third-Party Observation vs. Self-Observation

In self-observation, one observes his or her own actions or thoughts in certain situations. This approach can lead to invaluable information for professional development, supporting a reflexive practice in a systematic way.

Guidelines for Documenting Systematic Observations

Similar to other data collection methods, the success of the systematic observation in acquiring valid and reliable data depends on the quality of documentation of the observed events. In the following example, important background information is provided that will set the stage for introducing documentation guidelines. The approach uses multiple observations and is participatory, indirect, less structured, obvious, and in a natural setting.

> *Example.* Ellen is a teacher working with a special education program for children with learning disabilities. She has observed one student named Michael for three lessons to document and track his academic performance and learning. She videoed the lessons. Her observations from the first lesson are documented in the following report.
>
> *September 18, 2020: School's bakery practice session, 1st–5th periods, 8:10–11:50 a.m.*
>
> - Michael works with Frank during the baking session. Michael is responsible for making the dough.
> - Michael is easily distracted by Frank. Michael stops working and reacts every time Frank makes a comment.
> - Michael voices his opinions without needing much provocation. There is occasional laughter in the room, and every so often Michael will stop working and express his frustration.

- Frank is not distracting Michael on purpose, but he seems to like eliciting his reaction.
- Michael and Frank occasionally exchange jokes and pleasantries.
- Michael stands next to Victor during the kneading process. Victor is also good at interrupting Michael's concentration and winding him up.
- The kneading machines are placed in front of the window. Michael talks about what goes on outside and amuses Victor.
- Michael doesn't pay attention to the dough, which is getting dry. He eventually notices and corrects the problem.
- Frank finds the situation extremely funny and starts laughing at him. Michael tells him to "shut up."
- Michael seems to do well when he is focused on what he is doing.
- Michael works carefully and tries to avoid making mistakes. He carefully shapes the dough and brushes the egg wash on the top.
- Eventually, Frank makes another comment to provoke Michael. Michael becomes furious and starts yelling in the bakery, but they shortly start laughing again. After that, he goes back to the task at hand.
- Michael works hard to demonstrate his ability and carefully follows the instructions.

Guideline 1: Clarifying the Objectives and Areas of Observation

In the example of Ellen, the observation task was clear: observe one single student for three lessons. However, it was not indicated what specific (type of) behaviors she was supposed to observe. When you decide to perform an observation, it is important to carefully consider and plan important details of your observation related to the subject, the behaviors or activities, and the benefits of the observation according to the objective. This is relevant for both structured and less-structured observations. Based on this information, choose your desired areas of observation and list them in an observation chart. Ellen's areas of observation are not clear, which can pose a problem on the replicability of her observations.

Guideline 2: Documenting the Setting of the Observation

Ellen's note starts by describing the setting and writing down the location, date, and time of the observation: a practice session in the school's bakery on September 18, 2020, from 8:10 to 11:50 a.m. Make sure that all your audio and video recordings also start with this same information.

Ellen could have described the situation better by including additional details, such as the number of students attending the session, the layout of the bakery, the existence of major equipment, and the training objective. By describing the relevant context of the observation, you provide a clearer picture so others can better understand and replicate your experience.

Guideline 3: Describe Observable Verbal and Nonverbal Events Without Interpretation

Like any other data collection activity, the purpose of the observation is to collect raw data that you can see and hear. Therefore, your job as an observer is to only record verbal, nonverbal, and physical phenomena that could be observed. Ellen's report is not in compliance with that rule. Instead, she occasionally elaborates on previously observed behavior (e.g., "Michael voices his opinions without needing much provocation. There is occasional laughter in the room, and every so often Michael will stop working and express his frustration"). Furthermore, Ellen's report often contains her personal opinions and interpretations of the situation (e.g., "Frank is not distracting Michael on purpose, but he seems to like eliciting his reaction").

Some of the potential biases that can happen during observations include projection, subjective interpretations (e.g., taking position, making judgments, expressing sympathy), and stereotyping on the part of the observer (Ponte, 2002).

Projection: to place your own character, traits, desires, logic, and motivations on other people.

Subjective interpretations: to allow feelings of sympathy, dislike, or judgment toward a subject cloud your observation.

Stereotyping: to be influenced by a generalized image about certain groups of individuals. This may lead to prejudice, which means that you form an opinion about observed behaviors of members of a group that is not grounded in evidence.

In structured observations, you need to be mindful of how you choose your focal points relevant to the objective of the observation. The choice of focal points is always dependent on how the observer understands the phenomenon she is observing.

Example. A supervising staff member visits a shelter for victims of domestic violence to observe a support group session. She intends to observe which interventions the facilitator uses to stimulate the interactions between the participants. She uses the following chart to quantify the number of interventions in one session:

Focal points	Number of events
Facilitator asks clarification	4
Facilitator gives information	8
Facilitator invites participants to react to each other	3
Facilitator asks probing questions to guide the discussion	5

The focal points in the left column are regarded as actions that can help stimulate interactions between the participants. However, one can argue whether they actually can. For example, some actions may only stimulate interactions between the facilitator and the participants.

Guideline 4: Describe Triggering Factors in Less-Structured Observations

Behaviors often happen as the result of certain triggering (stimulating) factors. It is important to document the triggers immediately preceding the behavior in order to draw appropriate interpretations. In Ellen's example, she has described various conditions that triggered Michael. But her descriptions could include more details about what exactly happened (e.g., the nature of Frank's comment that provoked Michael). A more detailed description could have been:

> Frank says: "Hey, Michael, that's stupid!" He pointed to the way Michael was brushing the egg wash and that provoked Michael to yell at him.

The observation can be enhanced by specifying the exact timing of certain events (time stamps). Since Ellen did not use time stamps, it would be hard to accurately recreate the sequence of Michael's actions and their triggers.

Developing Observation Charts

Observation charts can be used during less- or more-structured observations. They often contain numerical, open-ended, and closed-ended areas of observation that are drafted in statement or question formats:

Numerical Areas of Observation: Examples

On average, how much time do the participants spend on completing the evaluation form?

How many questions did clients ask during the training session?

Closed-Ended Areas of Observation: Examples

Single-response areas of observation

Did the physical therapist review her notes from previous sessions at the beginning of the new session?

- o Yes
- o No

Multiple-response areas of observation

What teaching strategies did the facilitator use in the class?

- ☐ Group the participants based on their knowledge
- ☐ Create tiered modules
- ☐ Include practice exercises and projects
- ☐ Foster students' interests
- ☐ Practice flexible group activities

Scaled areas of observation

"The job coach helped his clients with their job searches and applications."

Completely agree   1   2   3   4   5 Completely disagree

Open-Ended Areas of Observation: Examples

What are the reactions of the Alzheimer patients living in the nursing home to the new navigational signage?

What topics do the patients often discuss with their dentists?

The instruments used in less-structured observations are similar to a logbook that contains open-ended areas of observation, which often includes the objective and the topics of interest (table 5.7). The following example also illustrates a less-structured observation approach:

Example. A group of social work students conducts an environmental scan of public places where prostitution activities are likely to occur. They create a map of parks, train stations, and shopping centers. They write down specific characteristics of each location a well as the type of activities related to prostitution, peak periods, and police presence.

Table 5.7. A log containing open-ended areas of observation

Date: Thursday, November 21, 2019

Time: 9:00–10:00 a.m.

Participants: Elderly nursing home residents diagnosed with early dementia

Activity: Participating in a vocabulary bingo game

Rules: Participants are supposed to fill in the blank squares on their bingo cards with vocabulary words to form complete sentences

Setting: Participants are seated in a circle

Objective: To form a clear picture about the type of behaviors that may indicate "patient engagement"

Notes: The observation was performed during my own group activity. I wrote down some examples of behaviors that I believe indicate patient engagement.

Time	Behavior indicating engagement
9:16	Participant B raises his hand and asks about the bingo process
9:18	Participant M covers his cards
9:20	Participant B laughs and yells that it is her turn to fill a square
9:22	Participant Z enthusiastically shows me her half-full bingo card

Depending on the objectives, there are four common observation instruments that could be used in structured observations (using close-ended or numerical areas of observation, adapted from Stokking, 2000):

Observation chart for monitoring the *occurrence* of particular events

Observation chart for monitoring the *frequency* of particular events

Observation chart for monitoring the *duration* of particular events

Observation chart for monitoring the *intensity* of particular events

Observation Chart for Monitoring the *Occurrence* of a Particular Event

This type of observation chart is used to verify whether certain behaviors or events occur in professional practice. The frequency and duration of the events are often not at the focus. Prior to the observation, you must define the characteristics of the observed event or behavior. You can subdivide the observation time into smaller units and tally the event at each of the time slots. In this way, you can document the sequential occurrence of the events.

Example. A therapist observes his performance during an intake interview based on a video recording. He tallies his specific actions in one-minute intervals throughout the interview.

Therapist actions	Interval in minutes					
	0–1	1–2	2–3	3–4	4–5	5–6
Asks open question	X		X			
Asks closed question		X				
Listens to the responses			X	X		
Explains the process				X	X	
Summarizes the key points					X	X

The tally shows the succession of the therapist's actions during the intake interview. It doesn't matter whether the actions occurred more than once per minute.

Observation Chart for Monitoring the *Frequency* of Particular Events

This type of observation chart is for tallying the frequency of various categories of behaviors.

Example. Lillian is an after-school teacher. Her supervisor has asked her to observe the children from the beginning to the end of playtime. Her job is to document the frequency of requests for guidance from the children, conflicts among the children, and the grievances of the children. She creates the following observation chart to tally the above areas of observation.

Time intervals	Requests for guidance	Conflicts	Grievances
During the introduction of the play activity	IIII	II	I
During the play activity	II	IIII	
During the conclusion of the play activity	II		I

The tallied observation provides useful information on how to allocate resources during different phases of play activities.

Observation Chart for Monitoring the *Duration* of Particular Events

This type of observation chart is used to document the duration of specific events and behaviors.

Example. Mark wants to assess the duration of patient activity during physical therapy sessions. He believes that most of the time in sessions is spent on communication and passive instruction rather than on actual exercise. He would like to verify his assumption by tracking how time is spent during sessions. To achieve that, he uses the following observation chart and a timer to tally each form of activity.

Duration	Exercise	Nonexercise
0–10 sec.	X	
10–30 sec.		X
30–55 sec.	X	
55–85 sec.		X

Observation Chart for Monitoring the *Intensity* of Particular Events

This type of observation chart is for assessing the intensity or quality of a situation or an event and is composed of *rating scales*. This is particularly useful, for example, when you are assessing the degree of adherence to a protocol, level of satisfaction with different components of a program, and/or quality of implementing subcomponents of a program. The chart usually includes scales based on subjective judgement about the intensity of an observed event.

Example. A supervising parole officer conducts a training workshop for his staff on drug use prevention. The goal is to reduce drug use–related violations of parole by creating awareness around triggers, helplines, available peer-support groups, and consequences of drug use. The officer is observed by one of his colleagues using the following observation chart:

Observation Chart: Drug Use Prevention Workshop					
The following components of the training are well designed and implemented:	Less than satisfactory	Satisfactory	Above satisfactory	Good	Excellent
Structure					
Sufficient and informative introduction				X	
Choice of topics covered				X	
Logical flow of topics					X
Timing and duration			X		
Summary and conclusion				X	
Technique					
Interactions with participants	X				
Effective teaching methods				X	
Use of technology			X		
Content					
Relevance to the needs of parole officers	X				
Depth and scope of the information		X			
Degree to which the information is up to date				X	

Exercise 1. **Logbook** (see page 169)

Exercise 2. **Observation Biases** (see page 169)

Exercise 3. **Less-Structured Observation Reports** (see page 170)

Exercise 4. **Assessing Patient Engagement** (see page 170)

Exercise 5. **Assessing Cross-Cultural Understanding** (see page 171)

5.4. Interviewing

Interviews are usually based on verbal questions that are asked in a personal conversation with the participants. Flick (2014) broadly describes two forms of interviews: semi-structured vs. narrative. Each form is distinctly different and requires a separate preparation strategy. Semi-structured interviews are conducted based on previously formulated written questions, while in narrative interviews, respondents speak freely in response to an initial open-ended question (probe) (Van Biene et al., 2012). Interviews must be planned ahead of time, but how and when questions are asked is dependent on the flow of the conversation and the type of interview. For example, you can request more information about something that the person just expressed ("Tell me more about what you liked about the center's parental support classes"). Narrative interviews are usually not interrupted unless clarification is needed or the response of the participant diverges widely from the topic of interview.

Interviews can be conducted individually or with a group of participants (group discussion or focus group). The selection of each method depends on the purpose and the nature of your inquiry. Individual interviews are more appropriate if you are interested in the experience of individuals, if you need to solicit in-depth input on sensitive topics, and when the confidentiality and privacy of your participants is a major concern. Group interviews are more appropriate when you are interested in the experience of a group of people, how a group of people interacts, or questions related to the culture of the group. In group discussions, participants influence each other, and this is useful for observing group dynamics and for finding out how a group discusses an issue.

Example. John is a youth counselor and his research is on bullying among children who participate in his support-group program. He found out that bullying has been a common practice in one of his groups. John decided to individually interview a few children from that group to learn more.

The reason for preferring the individual interviewing approach over a group interview in this example is based on the concern that a group might not be a safe place for the victims of bullying to fully express themselves, resulting in their being bullied during the interview. Also, peer pressure may influence children's responses toward more socially desirable ones. If so, the results would be unreliable. Further, a group interview in this case may aggravate the existing problems of bullying by raising awareness without offering solutions.

Interviews can be scheduled at any designated location, but you may find it easier to initiate conservations in natural settings where people work or receive services. For example, you can save more time by conducting short exit interviews or talking with a colleague/patient after a team meeting or during a treatment session.

Example. A juvenile justice center has launched a practitioner research study to learn about potential strategies for enhancing parental participation in the program. As a first step, the counselors are tasked to conduct 30-minute group interviews with the adolescents on this topic questions during their weekly group sessions using prepared questions.

In this case, conducting the interviews during regularly scheduled activities is a good choice, eliminating the need for planning a separate session for group interviews.

When possible, group interviews are usually more desirable for the following reasons:

Time commitment: Conducting several individual interviews requires significantly more time and effort than conducting one group interview with the same number of people.

Group dynamics: Participants' interactions in a group discussion provide interesting insights into how and why they react to various concepts and ideas.

Triangulation: Hearing participants' different perspectives and positions on a topic is a unique opportunity for considering a subject from different angles and thus for making a more differentiated assessment of the underlying problem.

Complexity of the topic: Most practitioner research topics are multifaceted and complex. Sometimes it is only possible to gain a full appreciation of this complexity in the context of a group discussion among a diverse group of participants.

During interviews, some nonverbal communication cues such as a participant's posture and physical expression can provide significant insights into understanding the practice problem. For example, a participant nods and shows signs of agreement during the conversation. Interviews can be influenced by the presence of other people, too (including you). Our spontaneous behaviors are often different from what we would like others to see. In the presence of unfamiliar faces, especially those of people in positions of authority, we may subconsciously start engaging in more socially desirable patterns of behavior. This is also the case when we are urged by others to show sympathy or antipathy toward an opinion or unresolved conflict; our reaction may not reflect our true opinion. The presence of an agency board member, for instance, may affect the answers of agency employees to questions related to workload.

You need to be mindful of the location where the interview takes place because it can significantly affect how people answer the questions. For example, interviews with employees on a topic related to work conditions that are conducted in a messy and poorly maintained room in a care facility may negatively affect participant responses.

Selecting or Developing Interview Questions and Guides

Similar to other systematic inquiries, you need to use valid and reliable interviewing instruments (interview guides) to ensure the integrity and replicability of your study. As discussed before, such instruments can be more or less structured, depending on the type of interviewing approach (semi-structured vs. narrative). In addition, you often need instructions as a supplement to the instrument to facilitate the interview process. The instructions are used by the interviewers to learn how to utilize the instrument and ask the questions according to a predetermined logical flow and sequencing. All three types of questions (numerical, open-ended, or closed) can be asked during an interview, and the technique for asking each type of question should be described in the instructions. Here are a few examples of each type of interview question you can include in your interview guide, followed by elements to include in your interview instructions:

Numerical Interview Questions: Examples

How would you rate the organization's overall influence on a scale of 1–10, with 1 being the least influential and 10 being the most influential organization in the field?

How many years have you been working as an occupational therapist?

Closed Interview Questions: Examples

Single-response questions

Check the box for the statement that you most agree with:

- ☐ I prefer house calls over parent meetings at the juvenile detention center.
- ☐ I prefer parent meetings at the juvenile detention center over house calls.
- ☐ I have no preference for either parent meetings at the juvenile detention center or house calls.

Multiple-response questions

What professional development activities are you interested in exploring to advance your career as a health educator in the next few years?

- ☐ New teaching methods, training methods, and technology
- ☐ Assessment and evaluation
- ☐ Partnership and interdisciplinary collaboration
- ☐ Grant writing and capacity building

Rating questions

I feel comfortable talking with my colleagues and asking for advice on issues related to patients' treatment and services.

Completely agree   1   2   3   4   5   Completely disagree

Open-Ended Interview Questions: Examples

What kind of language barriers did you encounter, if any, during the patient intake?

What do you consider to be a better approach for putting bullying on the agenda as a high priority topic in the nursing home?

The interview guide instructions should contain the following elements:

Description of the objectives for the interview

Documentation methods (e.g., note-taking, audio/video recording)

Ethical considerations regarding the privacy and confidentiality of participants, the interviewing process, data analysis, and dissemination of the results

Semi-structured interviews often follow a predefined logical outline with questions ordered accordingly. The logical flow of an outline is usually decided based on the type of study and the research question. By conducting a pilot interview before you begin your study, you will be able to determine if the structure you have created is appropriate. You can create logical outlines for your interviews based on one or a combination of the following approaches:

Functional: First start with participant backgrounds and experiences, followed by discussing their current roles, expectations, future plans, intentions, and recommendations.

Strategic: First ask about a participant's vision, mission, and strategic goals, followed by discussing practical actions and their significance.

Situational: First discuss the current situation, followed by exploring possible explanations, assumptions, and solutions.

Quizzical: First discuss what the issue is, followed by exploring why it has happened and how it can be addressed.

Chronological: First start with historical experiences and individual stories, followed by discussing their natural courses, the outcomes of different interventions, possible conclusions, and lessons learned.

It is always a good strategy to start with less sensitive topics until the conversation is warmed up and participants are feeling more comfortable, discussing more sensitive and controversial issues later in the interview. This can be done by first asking common questions about who they are and soliciting participants' general thoughts and opinions, followed by gradually probing deeper into more central topics of interest. This is also known as a funneling approach (or as a *funnel structure*). Alternatively, a *reverse funnel structure* (Bartelds et al., 1978) can be used as a strategy when you choose to start from details and progress to more generalized statements. In the next example, a few detailed questions are asked first, and the responses are revisited at a later stage in the conversation with a broader perspective in mind.

Example. You are conducting interviews with patients of a hospital about their general perception of safety and security. You start with specific questions related to their personal experiences in the hospital when navigating the building and interacting with fellow patients, as well as any concerns they have about the possibility of acquiring new diseases. As you move forward in the conversation, you probe into their perceptions of safety in each situation followed by a final request to make a generalized assessment of their overall sense of security in the hospital.

In a narrative interview, you generally start with a single question with areas for potential probing. Based on the problem definition and relevant theories you have discovered in the literature review, you can generate a list of main topics to initiate the interview (Boeije et al., 2009). Such topics can frame the discussion, but you still need to create a list of stimulating and probing questions to trigger and direct the conversation toward important details (table 5.8).

In your interview guide, you should also anticipate unusual situations and prepare questions to keep the interview on track. For example, in a situation when a participant starts complaining about something irrelevant, the interviewer can bring his attention back by asking questions that can guide the discussion to a relevant point or

Table 5.8. A qualitative interview guide in development		
Purpose of the interview	**Interview topics**	**Probing questions**
To deeply understand how my colleagues support the clients who have lost a loved one.	Grieving phase	Can you sketch phases (stages) of the grieving process using a practical example?
		What are the general characteristics of each phase?
		Tell me more about the first phase?
	Type of support	Can you describe a situation in which you have been able to support a client well?
		What forms of guidance do you use?
	Roles and responsibilities	What influence can you exert on the grieving process?
		What is the role of the relatives?
		What can the client can do for herself?
	Complex situations	Can you describe a situation in which you did not know how to act?
		Why was the situation complex?
		How did the problem start?

request postponing the discussion about the nonpertinent issue to a later time after the interview is completed.

Structuring an Interview Guide

A typical interview usually consists of three parts: introduction, central discussion, and conclusion. An interview guide can be structured around these three parts.

Introduction

During the introduction, basic elements of the interview are described, such as the objectives and rationale, the process, and the duration of the interview. It is the interviewer's responsibility to make sure that participants clearly understand the information about how the collected data will be used and seek permission for taking notes and recording the session. The process should allow enough time for participants to ask questions and become familiar with the process at their own pace.

Central Discussion

The most important part of the conversation occurs after the introduction and before the conclusion. This is the time when interview questions related to the main research question are asked. You need to be proactive and develop a set of questions and specific instructions on how to handle challenging situations. Interview and survey questions should contribute to answering the research questions.

Example. Wanda conducts short interviews with asylum seekers served by her center. This is part of a small study to better understand the needs of asylum seekers and their satisfaction with services. The questions that Wanda asks are about the residents' knowledge of their rights and responsibilities, asylum rules and regulations, their need for social activities, as well as their cultural beliefs and the political situations of their home countries.

In this example, not all of the questions are relevant to the objective of the study. This is something that Wanda should have considered and checked prior to conducting the interviews. Here are a few examples of common research objectives and appropriate questions for each:

To create a new service or intervention

- What are the interests of the target group?
- What interventions can help clients better reach their goals?
- What types of content should be provided?
- What roles can nurses play in providing the intervention?

To solicit participants' feelings and perceptions

- How do you feel when a patient is aggressive toward you?
- How do you feel when your opinion is (largely) ignored?
- In which parts of the neighborhood do you feel unsafe?

To solicit opinions

- How friendly have the staff and providers been toward you?
- What are some of the specific areas in which patients should have had a more prominent voice?
- How do you feel about the overall quality of supportive services for patients in drug recovery programs?

To explore ideas, real-world examples, and recommended solutions

- How can we improve the effectiveness of services? What would it take to achieve that goal?
- How can we build and maintain a better relationship with local residents?

To assess knowledge and skills

- Name two important signs of alcohol abuse.
- How many minutes will it take before the oxygen tank is depleted?

Avoid questions that suggest the desired answer. This might seem obvious and unnecessary to mention, but sometimes we use suggestive questions without intending to do so. Some examples of common interviewing problems are related to participants' misunderstanding of the questions, having a different expectation about the objective of the research, and interrupting the flow of the conversation by making comments that are not within the focus of the discussion at that moment. Such problems can be addressed more effectively when you have planned for them. In addition, you need to review the instructions and take time to prepare yourself for asking clarifying questions, probing confusing concepts, resolving potential misunderstandings, soliciting feedback, and asking follow-up questions.

Conclusion

At this stage, you give participants the opportunity to make comments or draw conclusions about the conversation. Describe your own impression of the results and reiterate the ways that you intend to use the data and knowledge gained from the conversation. Make sure to obtain an additional informed consent if you have new ideas about using or sharing any specific part of the information discussed during the interview. Lastly, this is a good time to explain how you will provide feedback on results of the study and thank the participant(s) for their time and input.

Questioning Techniques

Of course, not all situations can be predicted and addressed ahead of time. Therefore, there are special questioning techniques that you can use during interviews to improve your facilitation and problem-solving skills. Kvale (1996) describes nine techniques for initiating and facilitating interviews using different types of questions. In his approach, silence also has an important role and is emphasized as an effective way for not interrupting certain conversations and letting them take their natural course. You can choose among these techniques based on your personal taste and the context of the interview.

Opening Questions

Opening questions are usually broad enough to allow participants to start a conversation according to their own preferences and provide information they believe to be most important. This can spontaneously provide the interviewer with valuable insights about the participants' preferences and level of readiness to engage. In the course of the conversation, the information that participants provide could be further explored. Examples could include:

Tell me about . . . ?

Do you remember an incident where . . . ?

Can you describe a situation with sufficient amount of details where patients participated in the treatment process?

Follow-up Questions

Follow-up questions are asked to encourage participants to provide more details or tell us what they meant. A skilled interviewer continuously assesses the importance of certain information relevant to the objective of the interview. Zooming in on particular themes can be achieved in different ways, such as asking direct follow-up questions, repeating certain phrases, making short pauses, nodding, and/or expressing interest. Examples include:

You just mentioned . . .

Can you tell me what tools you used for that activity?

Can you explain what you meant by saying "I don't think my colleagues are well prepared for this"?

Probing Questions

Probing questions are used when interviewers want to delve into an in-depth discussion on a topic in an unbiased way. If done correctly, participants often voluntarily provide you with more in-depth information without getting an impression about the importance and desirability of any particular aspect of their responses. For example:

> Could you elaborate on that?

> Can you give me any other examples?

Specifying Questions

Specifying questions are asked to obtain further information to better explain a situation and/or provide more details about less clear terms and phrases expressed by a participant. Such questions solicit answers that help better specify and define ambiguous concepts, situations, and opinions using the participants' own vocabulary and examples. In other words, the answers to specifying questions help clarify what participants exactly meant by using a certain term, phrase, and label. For example:

> What did you mean by "empowerment"?

> How did you react when you realized that you were largely ignored?

> Have you experienced this yourself?

Direct Questions

Interviewers may choose to ask direct questions when they are in need of specific concrete details around an important topic or situation. It is best to save this type of question for when you have acquired substantial amounts of information and some gaps and missing details in your knowledge are identified. Some examples include:

> How frequently are peer coaching sessions held?

> You mentioned "evaluation" earlier. Were you referring to formative or summative evaluation?

> Have you been reimbursed for the cost of training?

Indirect Questions

Indirect questions are about acquiring information on how participants perceive other people's feelings, perceptions, behaviors, and reactions to a topic or a situation rather than making judgements about their own. Asking questions indirectly provides insights into participants' perceptions of social norms in a way that is less personal and therefore less anxiety provoking. For example:

> How do you think your colleagues perceive the quality of counseling provided to oncology patients?

> In your opinion, how supportive are nurses of the new patient education program?

Structuring Questions

Structuring questions (or comments) are usually asked when there is a need to direct the interviews along the planned outline and ensure that responses continue to generate relevant information. In addition, structuring questions help the interviewer to move on from one topic to the next. Examples include:

> Is it ok if we move on to the next topic?

> We have five more minutes left, and I would like to hear more about your personal experiences in peer support classes.

Interpreting Questions

Interpreting questions are asked to clarify ambiguous topics and validate the interviewer's understanding of responses. This can be done by repeating participants' answers using different wording (paraphrasing) or adding personal context (mirroring) and seeking participants' opinions to check their accuracy. Some examples include:

> Did you mean . . . ?

> Is it fair to say that you feel . . . ?

> Does the word "distrust" cover what you just described?

> Do I correctly understand that you think it is the management's responsibility to maintain a balanced workload?

> Am I correct if I say that the difficulties you experience with your mental health patients are somehow related to your low level of motivation to work with them?

> I get the sense that . . .

> If I understand correctly, you . . .

Silence

Silences and brief pauses can provide important opportunities for furthering the interview. They allow participants to bring their thoughts together, reflect on what they just said, and prepare for their next comments. But if they take longer than expected, you may want to break the silence to offer more information. The interviewer also can take advantage of this opportunity to review the conversation thus far and check if any topics have been overlooked. For example:

> The interviewer pauses for a few seconds and waits for the participant to answer the question.

> The interviewer stays calm and reflects on the participant's response, trying to fully understand it before saying anything further.

Logistics and Documentation

Health care and social work practitioners often have heavy workloads, so it is wise to plan your interviews with them well in advance. In addition, try to book a quiet, comfortable room and make sure that the duration of each interview is sufficient while not being too long. For many interviews, one hour to one and a half hours is sufficient. You may have to settle for less time in order to gain the consent of people with very full schedules. Participants often tell you at the start of the interview that their time is limited, but then they become so engaged in the discussion that they are willing to take more time than originally planned.

Make plans to record the session (audio or video). This will provide the best basis for your analysis. If that is not possible, decide how you are going to take detailed notes during the interview, including writing down direct quotations. Start each interview by documenting the name of the participant(s), date, time, and location of the interview. Also, make sure to document any special circumstances regarding the interview, such as working in tandem with other activities. Be sure to record the time the interview ended, too, so that you will know the duration of the interview.

Write the interview report promptly, while all information is still fresh in your mind. Audio or video recordings need to be listened to or viewed and transcribed as soon as possible. Transcribing a complete interview takes a substantial amount of time. Depending on the research question, you can choose to transcribe the whole conversation or only some parts of it. You may use the interview guide for analyzing the answers by grouping them under the interview themes and the outline. You may decide to validate the accuracy of your interview report by first sharing it with the participants and asking them to verify the contents.

Exercise 6. Planning and Conducting an Individual Interview (see page 171)

Exercise 7. Planning and Conducting Short Interviews with Patients (see page 172)

5.5. Surveying

Surveying is a more desirable approach when a practitioner researcher wants to quickly obtain information from a group of participants using either online or paper-based questionnaires. Survey questions, in contrast to interview questions, often are more restricted in their ability to allow for detailed clarification, probing, and follow-up questions. Sometimes participants are allowed to answer questions in their own words or to fill in the blanks, but the larger the group, the more the researchers should try to limit the use of such questions to reduce the time needed for completing the survey and analyzing the results. With smaller groups, however, it is more common and possibly more beneficial to include open-ended survey questions, since fewer responses means it will take less time to analyze the results. In addition, open-ended answers sometimes offer insights that you can further discuss in an interview. Two examples of cases when you may want to provide the participant with a less-structured way of responding are to (1) specify an answer to a question (such as the religious affiliation of the participant), or (2) provide feedback (such as information the participant thought was missing in the questionnaire).

Survey questionnaires can be self-administered using mail, email, or online surveying tools (e.g., SurveyMonkey, Qualtrics, etc.) or conducted at an in-person event where participants are informed about the process and can ask questions. Organizations may even choose to add their survey questions to an existing communication platform (e.g., newsletter, social media, website) to make the process logistically more convenient.

Example. Evonne is a nurse practitioner who works at a pediatric hospital. She wants to know how the patients' parents feel about the new design and color scheme of the hospital. After getting necessary permissions, she attaches a short questionnaire to the hospital's monthly online newsletter and asks the parents to participate in the survey.

Selecting or Developing a Survey Instrument

Developing a survey instrument can be a difficult task, and it is recommended that you only do it if no other relevant questionnaires exist. A questionnaire can contain numerical, open-ended, or closed phrases that can be written as either questions or statements.

Numerical Questions: Examples

How many minutes per day do you spend on bathing the patients in the ward?

How much do you weigh (in pounds)?

On a scale of 1–10, how do you rate the quality of the interactions in the discussion group?

You can also ask respondents to prioritize the answers by assigning descending or ascending numerical values to a set of predefined items. This is called a *ranking question*.

Example. Please rank the following topics for a smoking cessation support group based on your preference (1 is the topic that is most important, 5 is the topic that is least important).

Options	Ranking
Information about nicotine dependence	
Introducing and discussing nicotine replacement therapy	
Discussing participants' personal stories and their past attempts at quitting	
Engage in preparing a plan for quitting	
Providing information about nicotine withdrawal symptoms and triggers	

Closed Questions: Examples

Single-response questions

The respondent can only select one answer from the range of options.

Have you received treatment from this health care provider in the past?

☐ Yes

☐ No

Too many meetings are convened within the organization.

☐ Agree

☐ Disagree

☐ Neither agree nor disagree

Multiple-response questions

Check all the boxes that apply, indicating modifications made in your residence:

☐ Light switches at waist height

☐ Bath lift or shower stool

☐ Raised toilet seat

☐ Wall grip in the restroom

☐ Stair lift

☐ Electric door opener

☐ Other (please specify) _____

Rating questions

The therapy changed my daily routines and made me more physically active.

Completely agree   1   2   3   4   5   Completely disagree

Open-Ended Questions: Examples

How are the staff organized to provide meals at the center?

What are your ideas for involving fellow residents in activities?

Refining and Validating a Questionnaire

The questionnaire is a very important data acquisition tool that needs to be both valid and reliable. The overall effectiveness of a questionnaire is based on how the questions are written and ordered. Consider the following aspects (based in part on Bartelds et al., 1978) when you intend to write or choose the questions:

- If you will not be administering the questionnaire personally, it is important to provide a brief description of the research at the beginning. This includes the topic of the research, who is conducting it and why, and how the data will be used. There should also be a statement about anonymity, and it should clarify whom the participants can contact when they have questions about the research.

- Order the questions based on a natural and logical flow that makes sense to you and your colleagues. Document in clear terms information about the objectives of the questionnaire and how the data will be analyzed and disseminated. It is important for most respondents to know whether the survey is anonymous or not.

- Make sure that the options of (single and/or multiple) response questions are comprehensive to cover all possible situations. You can ask if the options are sufficient when obtaining feedback to a pilot test. Options such as "none of the above" or "other, please specify" provide the opportunity for giving feedback about unusual situations.

- It is often more difficult to analyze open-ended questions, especially if the answers are too abstract or ambiguous. Therefore, it is recommended to mostly use closed questions if you plan to survey large groups of people.

- Avoid using statements with double negative phrases, as these are harder to understand and you must take reverse reasoning into account when analyzing such statements. Examples to avoid include:

Why aren't you opposing the idea of not introducing the clients?

I do not unwillingly go to the daycare center.

    Completely agree   1   2   3   4   5   Completely disagree

- Organize the questionnaire by grouping together questions that have similar themes. When necessary, add instructions to each group of questions so respondents know what they are expected to do.

- A common problem when first designing a questionnaire is the tendency to ask too many questions. Bear in mind that having more questions elongates the time needed for completing the surveys and can adversely affect the accuracy of the responses.

- You can include the options "I don't know," "neutral," or "does not apply" in single- and/or multiple-choice questions to help the respondents who may not know the answer or find the options nonrelevant. However, selection of too many "I don't know" responses could indicate a lack of awareness or understanding of the topic in the target group.

- Participants occasionally select more than one option even when your questionnaire is designed to only allow for one single response. Indicating how many responses are allowed is very important. You may repeat this instruction with every group of multiple-choice questions. If you use computer-based questionnaires, you can often change the settings so that respondents can only select one option.

- You may structure a series of questions like a funnel. To do so, you may start with a general question on a particular topic and probe into more specific related issues in the subsequent questions.

- Filter (or contingency) questions allow respondents to skip those questions that are not relevant to their situation. For example, "If not, skip to question

X." If you use computer-based questionnaires, it is relatively easy to ensure that respondents automatically skip nonrelevant questions and follow question paths based on their answers to filter questions.

- Phrase the questions in clear and unambiguous terms to minimize misinterpretations and enhance the relevance and accuracy of the responses. For example, in the question "Are you involved with innovations?," it is unclear what innovations are being referred to, which aspects of the innovations are being focused on, and what exactly "being involved with" means.

- Is the question simple enough? Avoid using questions with complex words, a confusing sentence structure, or more than one topic. For example, "Can you specify what moved you to embark on a career in health care and how your journey started?" is actually two questions asked simultaneously.

- After writing the first version of your questions, share the questionnaire with your colleagues, patients, or other experts in the field before launching your survey. Ask several respondents or people that are otherwise representative of the target group to fill out the questionnaire and to give you feedback. This is called a *pilot test* or *pre-test* of the instrument. This helps you verify if the questions are worded and interpreted correctly. It also helps you measure how long it takes to fill out the questionnaire and whether more or fewer questions are needed. By going through this step, you can enhance the validity and reliability of your questionnaire.

- Consider any barriers potential participants may have when filling out your questionnaire and ways to overcome those barriers. This may mean increasing the font size or reading questions aloud when there is visual impairment, translating the questions into another language when participants may not read English well, adapting the language to the age or cognitive abilities of the participants, and/or incorporating visuals or props when administering the questionnaire (puppets, computer animation, color, or smiles to indicate levels on ranking questions, etc.).

- There are several online tools and resources for developing, distributing, and processing questionnaires. Some organizations often have subscriptions to survey design and implementation software for generating and distributing questionnaires. As mentioned above, computer-based questionnaires can save you considerable time for processing and analyzing the data.

Exercise 8. Designing a Questionnaire (see page 173)

5.6. Testing

Sometimes the research question is about measuring a participant's knowledge, attitudes, skills, or other characteristic on a given topic. In such cases, testing is the preferred method. Specific examples for testing in research include, but are certainly not limited to, verifying developmental or learning stages of participants, measuring the impact of a training intervention, monitoring the attainment of a skill (such as measuring blood glucose), and assessing levels of depression. Testing can be conducted by using standardized instruments, by designing your own interview or survey, or by making observations (such as using a checklist when participants are performing an activity). Specifically, when testing the acquisition of cognitive skills, the types of questions to be included can be assessed using the six levels of Bloom's taxonomy (Bloom, 1956):

Knowledge: being able to recite factual statements

Comprehension: being able to describe different variations in their own words

Application: being able to show mastery in a skill or competency

Analysis: being able to dissect a topic and describe its components

Synthesis: being able to create new forms of knowing and acting using the underlying concept

Evaluation: being able to reflect and assess a given situation and improve actions

Selecting or Developing a Testing Instrument

There are many standardized tests for measuring such personal characteristics as IQ, depression, activities of daily living, obesity, BMI, and the like. They are called "standardized" because they have been validated and often provide data that can be compared across different participants or assessments. They generally include instructions on how to perform and analyze the assessment, which may require a specific educational background for those administering the test. In some cases, you may have to ask an outside expert or a qualified colleague to assist you with choosing and/or adapting a testing instrument suitable for your target group, and to assist you in understanding the results.

You will have to design your own testing instrument if no appropriate tool exists for your objective. Dousma et al. (1997) have compiled the following general rules for designing a test of participants' levels of competency and knowledge regarding certain developmental or learning goals (and can be applied to designing testing instruments on other topics, as well):

- Clearly write down the objectives of the testing instrument.
- Align the questions or activities with their respective objectives.
- Formulate the questions or activities in collaboration with colleagues with relevant areas of expertise.
- Write the questions with careful attention to clarity and the specificity of the phrases; avoid using vague, confusing, and complex phrases.
- Provide a sufficient number of questions or activities for covering all the areas of interest.
- Allow enough time for completing the test.

Two types of questions or activities (open vs. closed tests) can be designed (Dousma et al. 1997). A closed test is comprised of closed and ranking questions. The possible responses to those questions are generally assigned a numerical value so that the answers of the participant can be added together to produce a score telling you, for example, how depressed the participant is or how able they are to conduct activities of daily living. Examples of closed tests include the following:

Yes/No Tests

A tablespoon of mayonnaise contains more calories than a tablespoon of ketchup.

☐ Yes

☐ No

Cognitive behavioral therapy is an effective treatment for dementia.

☐ Yes

☐ No

Multiple-Choice (Single-Response) Tests

How often do you have problems remembering appointments or obligations?

☐ Never

☐ Rarely

☐ Sometimes

☐ Often

☐ Very Often

Matching Tests

Draw lines between the columns matching the ranges on the left to the appropriate definition on the right:

0–12 months	School age
13–36 months	Infant
37–72 months	Preschooler
73–144 months	Toddler

The questions on open tests are open-ended and thus cannot be scored. This means that assessing open tests is more complex, requiring you to set clear assessment criteria beforehand. Types of open-ended tests include:

Oral Tests

Example. A counselor wants to assess the cognitive learning capabilities of a group of clients with mild cognitive impairment. He asks each client to study an illustrated brochure about the daily routine activities of a mailman. In the following week, the counselor schedules short interviews with the clients using a checklist to assess the knowledge they gained after doing the assignment.

Essays

Example. Compose a letter to the editor in which you comment on the upcoming policies stated in the institutional policy document. In your letter, specify what policies you either agree or disagree with, and why. You have a 500-word limit.

Short-Answer Tests

List three causes of high blood cholesterol.

Explain the meaning of the following sentence: "Market forces have a growing influence on the functioning of health care and social work systems."

Fill-in-the-Blank Tests

Dyslexia is also known as _____.

Red blood cells transport _____ and _____ in the blood.

Case Studies

Example. Adolescents read a fictional scenario about two boys having a conflict in school and are asked how they could more reasonably resolve the conflict.

Example. A group of family counselors discusses the following hypothetical case: You suspect serious child abuse in one of the families that you counsel. However, you do not have any concrete evidence or obvious signals to corroborate with your suspicion. What would you do?

Role-Playing

Example. A nursing supervisor asks his staff members who work in the emergency department to explain how they deliver bad news to patients. A guest actor is invited to role-play a patient so that the nurses can demonstrate their approaches. The results are analyzed to determine the strengths and weakness of current communication practices.

Practice Exercises

Example. Nursing staff are given an assignment on treating a simulation patient (with a specified illness) according to a specific protocol. They are allowed to use equipment that is present in the room.

5.7. Alternative Methods of Data Collection

In practitioner research, you often need to be creative and invent alternative methods of data collection, especially when you work with certain health disparities and disenfranchised groups of participants (e.g., poor, underserved, minority groups, people with disabilities). This is mainly because of such barriers as mistrust or perceived power imbalances that are hard to overcome through traditional methods of data collection. To bridge these gaps, you may want to bring your participants together in familiar and comfortable venues, such as outdoor events and festivals, churches, schools, and the like, where food is provided and people interact more naturally. In addition, you can enhance your participants' level of engagement in the research and increase their sense of ownership by using creative participatory methods, such as brainstorming, small group discussion, asset mapping, photography, and other active, entertaining activities. Research shows that visual and performance-based techniques are often more effective in engaging participants and attaining better learning outcomes (Wang & Redwood-Jones, 2001).

Selecting Alternative Methods of Data Collection

Alternative methods are usually qualitative in nature, focusing on the stories, experiences, and perceptions of respondents. This means that alternative methods of data collection generally result in less structured data, though you can use quantitative methods (e.g. a large-scale survey) in tandem. You may also still use such conventional methods as document analysis, observation, interviewing, surveying, or testing to collect your data but with more flexibility and a closer attention to the dynamics of the social settings in which you work. As with the data collection methods discussed in the previous sections, you can opt for an individual or group approach and you can apply the methods and techniques just once or several times. Following are a few examples of alternative methods of data collection, but remember you can always be creative and invent new forms of data collection that best suit your needs (see chapter 4).

Expressive Methods

Expressive methods are situations that can be illustrated by participants through role-playing, drawing sketches, or making short movies.

Example 1. As part of an in-service training at Child Protection Services, staff members are presented with a challenging case. Staff members are divided into two groups. After small group discussions, each group presents their recommended solutions through role-play. The facilitator writes down all the suggestions and thereby records ideas for resolving similar problems.

Example 2. A group of senior citizens participates in performing arts during their spare time. A student decides to investigate the impact of their engagement on their overall perceptions of well-being. This research question is explored with the use of improvisation techniques (i.e., casual conversations with probing) to urge the participants to reflect on their experiences and their impact.

Participatory drama, a particular expressive method, uses unique situations that could be best described through scenario-based role-plays or short movies followed by guided reflections.

> *Example.* Social workers in a child protection services agency are brought together for a practitioner research study to establish a common course of action for difficult situations where parents neglect the welfare of their children. The instructor divides the participants into three small groups. Each group is asked to discuss a case study and role-play the problems from different perspectives as well as the actions to be taken by the social worker to address them. All participants come together and share their experiences in a plenary session. All activities are video recorded for further analysis.

In this example, the case studies give the participants the opportunity to share their experiences relevant to the situation at hand. By role-playing, they actively engage in innovative ways to illustrate and solve the problem. Discussing the role-plays in the large group creates more opportunities for interactions, reflecting on ideas, and deepening understandings. Through video recording, the session can later be observed and transcribed, resulting in a richer analysis.

Visual Methods

Using images or objects to represent the practice problem and possible solutions is another alternative way to collect data. The use of visuals adds dimensions to the data that cannot be captured in words. Also, many people find it easier to visualize ideas than to verbalize them. And several visual methods (such as photovoice) engage participants in an activity that they find more enjoyable and interesting than discussing a topic in a group. Using images, particularly drawings, is very common in research with younger children.

> *Example.* A rehabilitation counselor would like to learn about his clients' preferred criteria for a new job. At the beginning of the session, the counselor covers the table with postcards and asks his clients to choose four cards that they associate with an ideal workplace. Then he asks his clients to reflect on their selection and explain why they made those choices.

In addition, images can help you improve your communication with patients for whom English is not their first language or who have difficulty verbalizing their ideas (such as younger children).

> *Example.* A nutrition and dietetics student charts the dietary habits of patients of Mexican origin whose English is limited. She uses a picture of food to aid in the discussion, in addition to working with a translator.

Photovoice is a technique through which you ask participants to answer research questions by taking photographs and writing down their comments. This photodocumentation method gives participants the option to document their health and work realities (Wang & Redwood-Jones, 2001).

Example. The findings of a neighborhood survey indicate that many local residents are worried about road safety in the area. The city council takes the matter seriously and plans to further investigate this issue. Thirty local residents are asked to photograph locations they believe would pose the highest risk of traffic-related accidents and draft their comments underneath their photos. At a subsequent meeting, the participants exhibit their photos and narratives at the city hall where legislators can view the exhibit, interact with the participants, and elaborate on their artwork.

Yet another method includes asking participants to create *3-D visual representations* of their opinions or concepts, either individually or as a group.

Example. Young residents of a dormitory are asked to create a model of their ideal living situation. They perform the task in pairs, using a variety of crafting materials. Upon completion of their work, the supervisor asks each group to fill out a form describing the primary features for a living situation they have illustrated in their models. The results form an inventory of recommended improvements for further developing the living environment in the dormitory.

Or ask participants to give a *presentation* on a particular theme:

Example. Patients in group therapy are asked to prepare a short slideshow about their favorite pastimes. The presentations paint an informative picture of the patients' leisure time activities for the group therapist.

Finally, *speech bubbles* are a technique wherein you present participants with a cartoon and ask them to imagine what each character is saying in their blank speech bubbles. This method is useful for visualizing the reactions of participants to certain situations that can then be discussed with other participants or with the practitioner conducting the study.

Example. A social work educator would like to know to what extent the students' attitudes about geriatric care are formed by their internship experiences. Prior to their internship, the educator asks the students to fill out blank speech balloons in cartoons depicting elderly patients in various situations in a hospital. Following the internship, the social work educator gives the same cartoons to the students and asks them to fill in the balloons. The educator asks each student to compare what they wrote before and after the internship experience and then facilitates a discussion in the group on what they have observed.

Narrative Methods

Storytelling can give researchers insight into people's feelings, experiences, and values in a unique way. By telling a story, the participant is able to share information about his or her experiences in a real-life context, as opposed to just answering questions. The discussion of stories enables people to compare their experiences and to reflect together on what those experiences mean in terms of addressing the practice problem under study.

One particular storytelling technique involves presenting participants with an unfinished short story and asking them to create the ending.

> *Example.* A social worker is providing counseling to a group of adolescents at a detention center. He tells the group several stories about everyday situations that present social conflicts. The participating youth are asked to finish the stories. This approach enables the counselor to gain insight into the lived experience of the adolescents as they have attempted to address conflict in their lives.

Story dialogue is another form of narrative data collection through which the participants recount events from their own lives in order to jointly find solutions (Labonte, Feather & Hills, 1999).

> *Example.* A school nurse provides an alcohol-use prevention training to middle school and high school students. To find out about the role alcohol plays in teenagers' lives, she encourages each group of students to tell stories of situations where drinking happens. Using the story dialogue method, the students then discuss each narrative in order to identify what using alcohol means in the life of the narrator. The group finishes their work by comparing their insights from each of the narratives to find the commonalities.

Participants can tell stories from their own perspective, or from a third-party perspective.

> *Example.* A public health counselor who works in a reproductive health clinic would like to understand the image that teenage girls have of Romeo pimps (human traffickers who usually operate by trying to make young girls or boys fall in love with them). Prior to the meeting, he asks the girls to write an entry in an imaginary sex trafficker's diary in which he tells the story of how he trying to recruit a young person into prostitution. During the meeting, the pages are read aloud, and the stories are discussed. Through this method, the counselor can form an understanding of how teenagers perceive Romeo pimps without having the girls discuss their own experiences publicly and explicitly. The stories are written from the perspective of another person, which allows the girls to draw from their experience or that of their friends without explicitly talking about it, thus protecting their privacy while providing a basis for a discussion on a sensitive topic.

Creative Thinking and Writing Methods

Mind mapping (described in section 2.3 as a way to explore a practice problem) can also be used as a data collection method:

> *Example.* An occupational therapist examines the effect of community meetings on the integration and social functioning of people with psychiatric problems. The community meetings are facilitated discussions between local residents and people with psychiatric problems who either live in the area or want to move back there upon discharge. Prior to the first meeting, the occupational therapist asks a group of psychiatric patients to create a mind map of how they see themselves integrating and interacting with others in the sessions. The patients are requested to review their mind map after participating in the meetings (three months after the start of the meetings and again after six months) to assess if their views have changed.

Journals are a good way to ask participants to record personal experiences and engage in self-reflection on the topic under study (see also section 2.2, technique 2). Journals often have a set structure that can be modified and adapted as needed. The structure helps participants capture the data more uniformly so the entries of different participants can be compared more easily.

> *Example.* A new program coordinator is responsible for organizing the first community engagement fair. She wants to keep detailed records of what works and what doesn't for future reference. Therefore, she asks the staff to keep a journal in which they note their daily activities and to reflect on the positive and negative aspects of each activity. The coordinator also asks them to note in their journals suggestions for improvement.

Decision-Making and Valuation Methods

You can stimulate participants to express their views by presenting them with *specific statements and hypotheses* and seeking their opinions:

> *Example.* You would like to learn about specific criteria that a team of therapists use for performing their work. You present the therapists with a brief case scenario and ask each member to describe what they would do in the scenario and why.

You could also ask participants to rate the statements with *scorecards* by assigning numbers or colors to each card:

> *Example.* A mental health care clinic investigates various ways through which the institution can effectively engage friends and family in the treatment process so the patients can better function independently in society. In previous meetings, several proposals were formulated and written on scorecards. The staff members are asked to individually rate the proposals during an internal workshop.

Lastly, a *nominal group* is a structured brainstorming session to reach agreement within a group on specific topics (Van de Ven & Delbecq, 1972). The structure assures that each participant contributes equally to generating responses:

1. Each member of the group individually compiles a list of three responses to the brainstorming question.
2. All group members present their responses, explaining the significance of their choices.
3. All the responses are combined into one list.
4. Each member ranks the top three responses from the combined list.
5. The rankings are then summed up to determine what the group, as a whole, finds to be the most important.

Example. A home care team leader wants to create an inventory of improvement strategies for the nursing staff. She schedules a few nominal group sessions with her colleagues to explore the following question: Which improvement strategies need to be incorporated in the center's internal policy document? They follow the structured brainstorming format so that the team leader gets ideas from everyone involved.

Measuring

Measurements can be taken with the aid of measuring tools, observation charts, performance tests, or questionnaires. Refer to relevant guidelines, protocols, and specialist literature if you plan to use measuring tools.

Example 1. A physiotherapist aims to improve reaction speed among her patients with brain injury. She uses specific therapeutic techniques and then utilizes tests to measure her patients' reaction speeds at the beginning, middle, and end of the study.

Example 2. "White coat syndrome" is a term used to describe patients' feeling anxious in the presence of the medical staff, resulting in higher blood pressure. A nurse practitioner wishes to establish if this is a problem among her patients. She gives blood pressure monitors to a few of her patients and asks them to measure their own blood pressure while at home. She will then compare the patients' self-measured results with the readings taken at the hospital.

Social Experiments

Certain social events and daily activities can provide good opportunities for conducting natural social experiments. The following classifications can be used as a basis for the preparation of an experiment (Van Lanen & Van der Donk, 2015).

Date, time, and duration: Indicate when your intended social experiment will take place and how long it will take.

Location: Describe where and under what circumstances the experiment will be carried out.

Participants: Identify the persons who will carry out the experiment or who will be part of the experiment.

Requirements: Make a list of materials, objects, and research instruments that are needed to carry out the experiment.

Sub-question: Write down the sub-question(s) that are relevant to your social experiment. Choose questions that are central to your experiment.

Expectations: Describe your expectation(s) about the possible outcomes of your experiment and their significance.

Arrangement: Provide accurate descriptions and take photos to depict the setting in which you want to carry out the experiment.

Process: Specify the steps you want to take. Your steps and processes should be clearly described so that others can replicate the experiment on the basis of your descriptions.

Data collection: Clearly indicate what data you want to collect during or after the experiment. Depending on the experiment you want to perform, you can decide to use one or more data collection methods.

Privacy and ethics: Ask the participants (or their parents/guardians) for permission to conduct the social experiment and take strict measures to protect participant privacy and confidentiality. Reflect in advance on possible effects and harms, if any, that the experiment might have on the participants.

Safety: Clearly indicate how you ensure the safety and security of the participants.

Example. A psychotherapist in a psychiatric clinic wants to find out if the size of the group affects patients' group participation. He believes that in a group larger than six persons, the participation is observably less. To test his hypothesis, the therapist creates groups of four, six, eight and ten participants. He writes down his observations regarding participation in his research journal.

Selecting or Developing Instruments for Alternative Methods of Data Collection

Most alternative methods of data collection are a derivative of methods that you use for document analysis, systematic observation, interviewing, surveying, or testing. You often use or develop instruments that are appropriate for the type of data you intend to collect, such as a comparison or observation chart, an interview guide, a questionnaire, a test, or a structured journal.

Exercise 9. **Developing Alternative Methods of Data Collection** (see page 173)

Similar departments, teams, or organizations are potential sources of valuable data and information related to your professional practice. Site visits allow you to observe and study various situations and also to interview or survey other practitioners so you can learn from their experiences.

Example. Marla has recently started her work as a music therapist, and she has the impression that her instructions are often too elaborate and complex for her patients. Her problem analysis shows that she uses only one instruction method for all her patients while there are new methods that might be appropriate for her sessions. To learn how to apply new forms of instruction, she decides to visit her fellow music therapy graduates who now work at different institutions.

If Marla just wanted to know what new forms of instruction are available, a literature review and/or discussion with senior colleagues would be sufficient. But she wants to see how to apply these new forms in a practice setting. A site visit provides that opportunity.

For each site visit, you need to specify the focus and objectives of your visit and prepare by creating research instruments relevant to the data collection methods that you want to use. In all, there is site visit preparation, the actual visit, and activities after the site visit to consider.

Site Visit Preparation

In planning a site visit, you need to first determine what site would be most relevant to visit and what type of visit would be appropriate. Answering the following questions can help with these decisions:

What is the objective of the visit?

What questions do I have that could be answered during the site visit?

When would be the best date and time for visiting the site?

Who should accompany me on this visit?

How long will the visit take?

What do I need to examine, observe, or study?

How should I collect the data (e.g., interviews, surveys)?

How will I use the collected data?

After completing this initial step, you can contact the place to request the site visit. The clearer you are regarding why you want to visit, the more likely your request will be granted. You need to clearly communicate about the data that you want to collect and the way that you intend to use that data. You also need to show respect and demonstrate understanding if the site you are visiting restricts what you can do on your visit (for instance, if annual reports are made available but not patient records).

After your request for the site visit is granted, there is still more preparation that you will probably do in cooperation with the site. Consider the following:

- Prepare a list of activities, a timetable, and expected results.
- Write down the contact information of key personnel from the site.
- Choose the most relevant methods for collecting data during your visit and create or refine the necessary tools and guides.
- Establish how the data will be recorded. You often need special permission if audio or video recording equipment is used.

The Actual Site Visit

Adhere to your planned timetable as much as possible but anticipate situations where the planned activities may need to be changed or revised. Keep in mind that you are a guest and will have to adapt to unexpected situations (e.g., unexpected events or activities taking longer than expected). To the greatest extent possible, try to be creative and make choices spontaneously that are aligned with the site visit objectives.

Example. Mary is a nurse working at the health department who is interested in learning about the experiences of Spanish-speaking patients at health care clinics. She decides to shadow a local team of health care providers for one day at a family planning clinic. She also plans to interview the providers and the patients after her visit. The shadowing takes longer than expected, and Mary has to choose between interviewing either the providers or the patients. As her objective is to learn more about the clinic's policy about communication with nonnative speakers and she has already spent a day with the patients, Mary decides to speak with the staff.

Following the Site Visit

It would be best to document your findings shortly after the visit, when all impressions are still fresh in your mind. Make every attempt to review, recollect, and add important relevant details that you observed or heard during your visit. If you were unable to document all the information at that time, read through the notes as soon as possible and add comments or information where necessary. You may want to color-code the additional notes to make it easier to distinguish the additions from the original notes at a later date.

Take the time to elaborate on the organizational context of the visited location. Indicate where and how the site's mission and context overlap with your own organization and where it diverges. It is courteous to share a copy of your report with the organization that you visited. You can ask the site for comments on your report, incorporate any critique into the final version, and thus enhance the validity of your research.

Selecting or Developing Instruments for Site Visits

The data collection methods that you can use during a site visit are similar to methods used for document analysis, systematic observation, or questioning. You may select already developed tools or design your own instruments, such as a comparison or observation chart, an interview guide, a questionnaire, a test, or a structured journal.

5.9. Summary

Several data collection methods were discussed in this chapter. Data collection is usually facilitated by using relevant tools, also called data collection instruments. These are, for example, comparison charts, observation charts, questionnaires, or tests. If no existing instrument is suitable for use in your study, you need to develop or adapt an instrument that meets your needs. The development of an instrument for data collection is informed by the practice problem, knowledge gained through the literature review, and the research question. Depending on the type of instrument, data collection tools often have specific components, such as focal points, areas of observation, and questions.

Textual sources can be analyzed by using a comparison chart with a list of focal points derived from the research objective to examine contents from internal and external documents. Having inclusion and exclusion criteria help you filter useful textual sources that you want to select for your research.

Observation can take such forms as single vs. repeated, participant vs. nonparticipant, direct vs. indirect, structured vs. less structured, natural environments vs. controlled settings (field vs. lab), and third-party vs. self-observation. Data from observations are often recorded in observation charts.

Interviews, surveys, and tests are commonly used data collection methods for acquiring information regarding the perceptions, experiences, knowledge, and skills of study participants. Interview guidelines help structure the interviews. Surveys are a form of interviewing via questionnaires. Tests help you gain insights into specific characteristics of your participants.

In practitioner research, you often need to be creative, inventing alternative methods of data collection. The methods may be adaptations of conventional methods or methods that are very different in form and type of data.

The initial considerations for planning a site visit are related to determining where to visit and why. Next, you want to consider how to carry out the site visit and other associated activities. Site visits require proper planning on how to identify and communicate with the site, clarify the contributions of the visit to your research, and design needed data collection methods and tools. Clearly communicate your plan for analyzing data and reach agreement on issues related to documentation and dissemination of the findings with the organization that you are visiting. Document your findings thoroughly and systematically in a report; be sure to describe the organizational context.

Exercise 1. Logbook

The learning center at a mental health clinic offers a group activity called Memory Café for elderly patients with early dementia. The goal of the group is to enhance the quality of informal care provided by the families of the patients by demonstrating how they can support the patients in their memory loss. A small number of informal caregivers are asked to keep a short log and document their experience.

Answer the following question: What would be a suitable format for the caregivers' logbooks?

Exercise 2. Observation Biases

When describing your observations, be aware of biases such as projection, distortion due to overidentification or disagreement, and stereotyping. Do any of the following biases sound familiar to you? If so, which ones? Add two more examples of your own to each type of bias given here.

A social worker has problems working with clients with addiction. He assumes that clients with addiction are unreliable and aggressive. (Stereotyping)

Peggy hated fieldtrips as a childhood. Peggy is pessimistic about the upcoming field trip as she fears that the children might not look forward to it. (Projection)

When she was younger, Maria was bullied a lot. During her internship in an after-school center, she notices that one of the children is very quiet and does not engage in play activities much. Maria keeps an eye on him and sees more and more indications of possible bullying. When the pediatrician examines the young student, he finds that the child is hearing impaired. (Projection)

The instructor is giving instructions about an activity. Suddenly, Martin shouts that it is snowing outside. The instructor looks and notices the first snowflakes of the season. He is fond of Martin and smiles. He continues with his instructions. John then loudly asks, "Can we go outside?" Other members nod and show their signs of approval for John's suggestion. The instructor, however, is irritated because John is a troublemaker, so he tells John to be quiet. (Distortion due to over-identification or disagreement)

Exercise 3. Less-Structured Observation Reports

Two observers simultaneously observe a patient leaving the activity center in an irritated mood. Compare the two resulting reports and mark the main differences.

Observation Report 1

1. John immediately starts preparing for his physical therapy treatment.
2. He packs his items in a couple of boxes.
3. He turns back and looks at the counselor after he finishes packing.
4. He turns around, watching other patients. He seems to be amused by what others are doing.
5. He says something to a patient about the items near him that were still on the table.
6. He turns back and talks briefly with his therapist.
7. He walks out the door.
8. He seems to be upset, and I found his behavior somehow exaggerated.

Observation Report 2

1. John is seated on a chair and he picks up a box.
2. He places his personal items in the box.
3. The counselor calls him by his name. John looks up.
4. Casey (the patient on the bed beside him) taps him on the shoulder. John turns around.
5. John says, "You should put that stuff in the box!"
6. The counselor tells John that it is okay to ask if he doesn't understand the instructions.
7. John turns back to the counselor and looks at her.
8. John says, "I know perfectly well what to do."
9. "I thought you were unclear about something," says the counselor.
10. John gets up, tosses the box on the floor, and walks out.

Exercise 4. Assessing Patients' Engagement

It is recommended that you conduct this exercise in pairs by making repeated observations of a patient or client during their participation in two group counseling activities. This exercise enhances your ability to observe and monitor each participant's unique signs of engagement.

1. Team up with a peer and jointly identify a client whose engagement you would like to observe. Identify your areas of observation, prepare a guideline, and design an observation chart. Refer to the literature for defining "engagement."
2. Separately, but simultaneously, observe the patient during two group counseling sessions and write the results in the observation chart. Describe the ob-

served situations and behaviors as accurately as possible. It is important that you perform and record your own observations independent from your peer.

3. When both observations are concluded, share and discuss your charts. To what degree did each of you follow the observation guidelines? What similarities and differences do you see in your chart? Do you have an explanation for those differences?

4. Examine and analyze your findings (see chapter 6) and consolidate your views about the patient's level of engagement in the process.

Note: Make sure that you communicate your plan with the patient and ask for his or her permission. It may be useful to share some of the insights that you learn with the patient after conducting the exercise.

Exercise 5. Assessing Cross-Cultural Understanding

Health care and social work professionals need to be culturally competent in addressing the needs of patients from different backgrounds and communicating with them effectively. Hoffer (2010) describes that merely knowing about a culture and/or religion, even though necessary, is not sufficient for an effective cross-cultural communication. A provider must develop a positive attitude toward learning other cultures and make conscious efforts to understand the realities and value systems of clients from diverse and minority backgrounds. The most important precondition to achieve such a goal is through actively listening to and asking questions about the patients' stories, opinions, feelings, and behaviors, without any prejudice or stereotyping attitudes.

The objective here is to practice your ability to observe a practitioner's interaction and communication with patients from a different cultural background than their own.

1. Talk to a practitioner and ask for her permission to conduct the observation (and ask for the patient's permission as well).

2. Describe the scope of your research using the literature and design an observation chart.

3. Observe the practitioner in a situation where she is providing care to a patient from a different cultural background.

4. Discuss the main points of your observation with the practitioner.

5. Examine and analyze your findings (see chapter 6) and formulate your view about the practitioner's cross-cultural communication approach.

Exercise 6. Planning and Conducting an Individual Interview

Health care and social work practitioners often encounter difficult and challenging patient situations. Some practitioners have the knowledge and communication skills for addressing most challenging situations while maintaining a professional relationship, but others may not perform as well in certain situations and become frustrated and exhausted. You decide to study this practice problem by exploring what kind of challenging cases practitioners face and how they usually handle these situations. The first step is to describe the definition of "a challenging situation." In order to do so, you want to interview several practitioners to find out when they consider a case "challenging" and why.

Prepare a guideline for a 10-minute individual interview for gathering data about the above practice problem using a few focused questions. To test the guideline, ask your colleagues to both participate in an interview and observe other interviews. Ask them to tell you their opinions about how to improve the process and make the questions clearer. Tell them to assess the clarity of the questions, any influences on responses to the questions, and the relevance of the questions to the interview's objective. You may want to use a simple chart similar to the one here to document the findings.

Interview observation chart	
Questions	Comments
Q1	Clarity:
	Influence:
	Relevance to objective:
	Other:
Q2	Clarity:
	Influence:
	Relevance to objective:
	Other:

Exercise 7. Planning and Conducting Short Interviews with Patients

Having well-planned short conversations with patients/clients is a good way to quickly get to know them and better understand their needs. The objective of this exercise is to self-assess your ability to plan and conduct a short interview with a small group of patients/clients. Perform this exercise with a peer, if possible.

1. Identify a group of patients/clients for the interview and decide
    a. the objective(s) for your interview,
    b. the questions you are going to ask,
    c. the cast of role(s), and
    d. the duration of the interview.
2. Prepare for the orientation and interviews by
    a. creating a simple informed consent and invitation process,
    b. blocking out the interview dates and times in your calendar,
    c. identifying and reserving a suitable location for the interviews, and
    d. planning the scheduling process.

3. Conduct the interview and take notes. Use recording equipment only if you have prior consent from the patients.

4. Write an interview report as soon as possible.

5. Discuss the following questions and write down your conclusions:

   a. Were you able to get the information you were looking for? If so, to what extent? If not, why not?

   b. What went well? What could be improved?

   c. To what extent did you follow the interview guidelines (see section 5.4)?

   d. How would you change your approach next time?

Exercise 8. Designing a Questionnaire

Design a questionnaire using a five-item Likert scale to collect data about the perceptions of staff on issues related to their working conditions and the organizational culture in the following scenario. The data will help the organization's board of directors to make improvements (see Exercise 9).

In a previous meeting, several staff members expressed discontent regarding the overall atmosphere as well as the organization's norms, rules, and policies. They were concerned that some staff members treat patients as they see fit, lacking consistency and integrity when it comes to the quality of care. The management designed a questionnaire to assess the staff's definition of the term "consistency and integrity." Steps may be taken to improve internal policies based on the results of the survey.

Exercise 9. Developing Alternative Methods of Data Collection

Select or develop an alternative method of data collection and work it out in such a way as to collect information that the management in the example of Exercise 8 can use it to make a decision about how to improve the working environment.

REFERENCES

Bartelds, J. F., Kluiter, H., & Van Smeden, K. G. (1978). *Enquête-adviesboek. Een handleiding voor het verzorgen van schriftelijke enquêtes* [Survey handbook: A guide to conducting surveys]. Wolters-Noordhoff.

Bloom, B. S. (1956). Taxonomy of educational objectives, vol. 1: Cognitive domain. McKay.

Boeije, H., 't Hart, H., & Hox, J. (2009). *Onderzoeksmethoden* [Research methods]. Boom Uitgevers.

Dousma, T., Horsten, A., & Brants, J. (1997). *Tentamineren* [Examining]. Wolters-Noordhoff.

Hoffer, C. (2010). Neem niet aan, maar vraag! Interculturele communicatie in de gezondheidszorg [Don't assume, but ask! Intercultural communication in health care]. *Phaxx*, *9*(1), 12–14.

Flick, U. (2014). *An introduction to qualitative research*. Sage.

Kvale, S. (1996). *InterViews: An introduction to qualitive research interviewing*. Sage.

Labonte, R., Feather, J., & Hills, M. (1999). A story/dialogue method for health promotion knowledge development and evaluation. *Health Education Research*, *14*(1), 39–50.

Ponte, P. (2002). *Onderwijs van eigen makelij* [Design your own education]. Nelissen.

Stokking, K. (2000). *Bouwstenen voor onderzoek in onderwijs en opleiding* [Building blocks for research in education and training]. Universiteit Utrecht.

Van Biene, M., Kohlmann, J., Heessels, M., Bobbink, E., Degen-Nijeboer, H., Geurts, E., Pelzer, M., & Woudenberg, J. (2012). *Narratief! Wablief? Ieder zijn eigen verhaal* [Narratives! What do you mean? Everyone his or her own story]. Hogeschool van Arnhem en Nijmegen.

Van de Ven, A. H., & Delbecq, A. L. (1972). The nominal group as a research instrument for exploratory health studies. *American Journal of Public Health*, *62*(3), 337–342.

Van Lanen, B., & Van der Donk, C. (2015). *Onderzoekend leren: Een stappenplan voor onderzoeksopdrachten* [Inquiry learning: A step-by-step plan for inquiry tasks]. Uitgeverij Van der Donk & Van Lanen.

Wang, C. C., & Redwood-Jones, Y. A. (2001). Photovoice ethics: Perspectives from Flint Photovoice. *Health Education and Behavior*, *28*(5), 560–572.

6

Analysis and Conclusion

Analysis is when the answers to research questions are extracted from the collected data and formulated into conclusions (figure 6.1). This chapter details those steps and contains general recommendations for both analyzing data and forming conclusions. Distinct processes of analysis for quantitative and qualitative data are included as well since these different types of data must be handled each in their own way. Lastly, a brief summary and relevant exercises conclude this chapter.

6.1. From Collected Data to Findings

At this point in the process, you will draw on the collected research data and formulate conclusions on the basis of your findings (figure 6.2). The following three steps will get you from raw data to general findings.

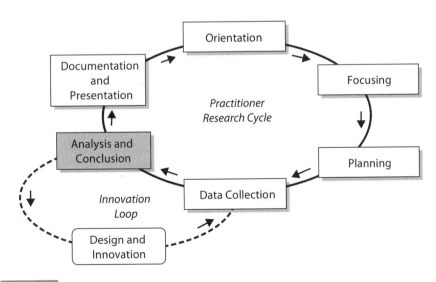

Figure 6.1

Key components of practitioner research: Analysis and Conclusion

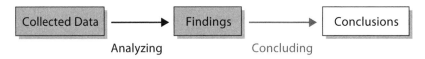

Figure 6.2

The analysis process turns collected data into findings

Organize the Data by Sub-Question

In the research plan, you specified which method of data collection you intended to use for each of the sub-questions. You may have used a single method of data collection (such as patient interviews) to answer several sub-questions. You need to sort this data collection according to the relevant sub-questions before starting the analysis (table 6.1).

Reduce, Combine, and/or Transform the Collected Data

Your research activities may yield a large amount of data, which will need to be reduced or summarized so that it is relevant, useful, and clear. Primary data needs to be separated from secondary data. In this case, the primary data is information that contributes to answering the research question and sub-questions, while secondary data does not. The process of refining the information is also called *data reduction*.

> *Example* 1. The care provided to inmates after their release from prison is examined in order to determine if the program needs to be modified. A team leader gathers a substantial amount of information by interviewing several experts, studying relevant literature, and talking to ex-detainees who have returned to so-

Table 6.1. Sorting data by sub-question before analysis begins	
Sub-question	Data that answers the sub-question
Which problems do aphasia patients experience daily when communicating?	Answers 3, 4a, 4b, 5, and 6 from the partner/family questionnaire. Points 2, 3, and 5 on the comparison chart from my literature review on aphasia.
What targeted forms of support do aphasia patients need in order to be able to make phone calls?	Answers given to questions 4 and 5 by the neuro-psychologists during the group interview.
Which medical tools or resources can be used to facilitate communication with aphasia patients?	Data related to points 1 and 4 on the comparison chart from my literature review on aphasia. Answers given to questions 1, 2, and 3 by the neuro-psychologists during the group interview.

ciety. The resulting large amount of data is overwhelming, so the team leader divides it into smaller parts. These parts are based on his research sub-questions that have three themes: housing, building a social network, and earning a steady income. The team leader organizes the data according to these themes, leaving out irrelevant information.

Example 2. The atmosphere in one of the residential groups at a boarding school is far from ideal. The group leader asks each of the youth in the class to write up their thoughts about the overall emotional climate of the group. She separates the data into four categories for her analysis, thereby giving her insights into what the youths mean by a "bad atmosphere."

Data reduction is often achieved through *transformation*, which makes the data more useful and more manageable. Transformation essentially means presenting information in another form(at) in order to gain better insight into the findings. The content of the data (and thus the research findings) should remain unchanged in this process. The leader in each of the examples above effectively changed the appearance of the data and thus *transformed* it from narrative answers into categories that could then be further analyzed.

Example. Cindy wishes to know how her home-care patients define her nursing approach. She gives each patient a list with 20 definitions and asks them to choose five terms that best describe her work method. Cindy transforms the raw data by tallying the frequency of each selected definition and subsequently calculating the resulting percentages. She presents these percentages graphically in a pie chart.

In this example, the data from all questionnaires is reduced by transforming them into numbers that can then be displayed graphically for the purpose of comparison.

Depending on the sub-questions, you will probably not only transform the data but also *combine* them. For example, you can compare answers from different subsets of respondents by linking the answers to age or gender. You can also combine data to depict progress. For instance, for a full year you can ask patients at the end of each week how much time they have spent with other patients. You can then combine these weekly datasets to chart the progress throughout the year.

You usually take into account your intention to reduce or combine data categories when designing your data collection instrument(s). Sections 6.2 and 6.3 present additional methods of analysis for data reduction, transformation, and combination.

Present the Analysis Results (Findings)

The analysis results (or *research findings*) are the part of the data that remains after you have organized, reduced, transformed, and combined the collected information. This remainder leads to the answers of your sub-questions and is presented in numerical, textual, or graphic format (such as graphs, pie charts, and infographics).

6.2. Analyzing Quantitative Data

The data gathered in practitioner research can take various forms. Quantitative data is strictly numerical (such as age or weight) or data that is easily converted into numbers (such as multiple-choice questionnaires).

Example. At the end of each workday, a job coach asks her clients to pick one activity (from a list of work activities) that they had the most trouble with on that day. She subsequently tallies the selected activities, thereby converting the data into numbers.

Statistics is a mathematical discipline that uses different operations to analyze quantitative data. There are two forms of statistics: descriptive statistics and inferential statistics. Descriptive statistics express the research data in frequencies or percentages of the total number of observations. These figures are often presented in tables, pie charts, and bar graphs. Descriptive statistics are sufficient when your research population, the group you want to study, is small. This is the case in most practitioner research projects. For example, you are conducting an evaluation of a small family counseling practice and you receive responses from all or most of your clients.

If, however, your research population is large—that is, you cannot reasonably include everyone in your study—you need to draw a *sample* to answer your questions. A sample is a subset of the research population that you choose to take part in your study. For example, you are conducting an evaluation for a large family counseling center which has served 3,000 families over the last two years and you are only able to reach 200 of those families with your questionnaire. In those cases, descriptive statistics are not sufficient, because the larger group may be quite different than the smaller group you have included. Instead, inferential statistics are used to infer or extrapolate results obtained from a sample to a much larger research population.

Inferential statistics uses correlation coefficients, chi-square tests, t-tests, regression analysis, and other methods to determine if the research results are statistically significant and thus likely to also represent the larger population and not only the sample. In other words, inferential statistics answer the following question: Are the sample results indicative of the results that would be achieved if the entire target group were included? Further resources on applying and interpreting inferential statistic can be found in well-known software programs such as Excel, SPSS, or GNU PSPP, and in the relevant literature.

Here we present several basic methods for analyzing quantitative data using descriptive statistics. The methods you use are dependent on the types of variables found in your data. A *variable* is a characteristic of the people (or other units) you are studying. These characteristics vary depending on the person, hence the name "variable." Why they vary—that is, why certain people have certain characteristics and others do not—is at the heart of social science research, including practitioner research. In general, each question in your study stands for a variable. The possible answers to the question are called *items*.

Examples. In practitioner research we often ask people if they belong to a certain group. If the question is "What is your profession?," then the variable is profession. We may give the participants choices: for example, social work, nursing, or physical therapy. In that case there would be three items. Or we can leave the question open. In which case the number of items would be the number of different professions given by the participants.

Another common question is about client/patient satisfaction, which is often asked by giving participants several choices for their answer.

How satisfied are you with our services?

☐ Very satisfied

☐ Satisfied

☐ Dissatisfied

☐ Very dissatisfied

The variable is client/patient satisfaction and there are four items.

Another common question in practitioner research is the age of the participant: "How old are you?" Age is the variable, and the items are the ages given by the participants.

There are three types of variables: nominal, ordinal, and interval. With nominal variables, the items are not in any hierarchical relationship to each other. That is, neither answer is somehow higher or lower, better or worse than the others. The profession variable above is nominal. Other common nominal variables are gender, religious affiliation, place of residence, or ethnic group.

With ordinal variables, the items are in a hierarchical relationship to each other. The client/patient satisfaction variable just mentioned is ordinal. On the high end is "very satisfied"; on the low end is "very dissatisfied." Other common ordinal variables are level of education, level of professional certification, or role in an organization.

The items in interval variables represent a quantity that can be measured exactly and the items have a mathematically exact relationship to each other. The age variable above is interval. Other common interval variables in practitioner research are years of professional experience, the amount of time a service is provided, patients' weights or vital signs, or measures of physical ability (such as number of steps walked or range of mobility). The relationship to each other can be expressed mathematically: Someone who is 10 years old is twice as old as someone who is 5 years old. Someone with 20 years of professional experience has five times the years of experience as someone who has been working for four years. In ordinal variables, this relationship is not exact. You cannot say that someone who is "very satisfied" with services is twice as satisfied as someone who checks "dissatisfied."

Appropriate methods for analyzing interval, nominal, and ordinal variables are described next, followed by a discussion about standardized tests.

Data Analysis for Interval Variables

Interval variables can be quite feasibly combined, as the values have fixed mathematical relationships to each other. It is relatively simple to verify which individuals or groups possess or display more or less of a certain characteristic, such as higher grades for students who prepared for a test compared to the students who did not prepare. Several different mathematical operations can be performed with such data.

Interval Analysis Method 1: Calculating the Average (Mean)

To calculate the *average* answer returned by all participants:

1. Sum all returned scores to a particular question.
2. Divide this by the total number of participants in the group. Exclude blank answers or unreturned questionnaires from the calculation.

Interval Analysis Method 2: Finding the Median

The *median* is a number that indicates the middle of a dataset, which can be calculated for both interval and ordinal variables. Averages can be strongly influenced by individual anomalous small or large values and may therefore lead to skewed results. For example, in a group of five individuals aged 8, 50, 65, 54, and 52, the average age is 45.8—even though only one of the members of that group is younger than 45.8. The same can happen, for example, when using average values for determining how much pocket money youths in a juvenile center receive from their parents or guardians: if one member of the group receives an inordinately high amount, the resulting average allowance does not correspond with most of the youths' realities. The median value, on the other hand, indicates the exact middle of the dataset: half of the values are above and half of the values are below the median. In order to calculate the median:

1. Place the data in ascending order.
2. Find the number in the middle (where there are an equal number of data points above and below the number).

Example. The group of five individuals already mentioned aged 8, 50, 65, 54, and 52, whose average age would be 45.8, looks a little different when solving for the median age:

Individual ID	1	2	3	4	5
Age	8	50	52 (median)	54	65

Note: If the dataset has an even number of data points, then add the two middle numbers and divide by two to find the median.

Interval Analysis Method 3: Finding the Standard Deviation

Standard deviation is a measure of dispersion that shows how the data is clustered around the mathematical average (or mean):

1. Determine the mathematical average, or mean, for all the answers.
2. Calculate the difference from the mean for each individual answer.
3. Calculate the square of each of those differences.
4. Determine the average of the resulting squares.
5. Calculate the square root of that average.

Example 1. Five participants complete a psychological test, for which the maximum score was 5 points. The participants' scores are 5, 1, 4, 1, and 4, respectively. The average score is 3. The differences from the mean are +2, −2, +1, −2, and +1, respectively. The squares of these differences are 4, 4, 1, 4, and 1, and the average square is 2.8. The square root of 2.8 is 1.67.

This means that the standard deviation for the five participants is 1.67, which is relatively high, given that there are only 5 points in the scale. The individual scores explain this fact, as they are divided in three high scores of approximately 4 and two low scores of 1.

Example 2. After weighing 30 participants, it is determined that the average weight is 159 pounds (lbs) with a standard deviation of +/−3 lbs. Most of the participants weigh between 156 lbs and 162 lbs.

The larger the standard deviation (difference from the mean), the more the individual values vary. A standard deviation of 0 means that no answers deviated from the mean and that the (average) score is the same for all participants. What constitutes a large standard deviation is based on the scale of measurement. Using our prior examples, on a 5-point scale 1.67 is a large number; whereas within the range of possible body weights, the standard deviation of 3 is small. You can only compare standard deviation values when you are measuring the same things.

Example. Thirty adolescents in two different residential groups are surveyed about their internet use. Group A averages 870 minutes per week, with a standard deviation of 252 minutes. Group B equally averages 870 minutes, but with a standard deviation of 20 minutes. The standard deviation of 252 minutes in group A is large compared to the average time spent surfing the internet (870 minutes), whereas the 20-minute standard deviation of group B is small. This is an indication of the large variance in the answers of group A.

For large amounts of data, it is nearly impossible to perform calculations of averages, medians, and standard deviations by hand. Software programs such as SPSS, GNU PSPP, and Excel are useful tools in such cases.

Interval Analysis Method 4: Comparing Numerical Data

Comparing numerical data and presenting the results in a different way can lead to new insights. Consider for example the following two questions from a questionnaire:

How many years have you been with the home care organization?

How many minutes per week are spent in contact with patients?

Comparing these questions may tell you whether there is an association between time spent with patients and the number of years that the nurses are employed by the organization. Certain visualizations of the data can aid such comparisons, for example, graphs, bar charts, and tables. These are easily generated by using software programs such as SPSS or Excel.

Exercise 1. Asking Questions with Interval Variables (see page 202)

Data Analysis for Nominal and Ordinal Variables

Nominal and Ordinal Analysis Method 1: Calculating Totals (Frequencies)

When you calculate totals (or *frequencies*), you are determining how often a particular option has been given.

1. List all responses (items).
2. Tally every instance of a particular response.
3. Add the tally marks per item.

Example 1. A physical therapist wants to know what time of day her patients prefer to do prescribed exercises so she can make the appropriate recommendations. Her question to her patients is, "Which is your preferred time slot for doing your exercises?" She calculates item totals using the following table:

Night (between midnight and 6:00 a.m.)   ℍ I   = 6

Morning (between 6:01 a.m. and 11:59 a.m.)   III   = 3

Afternoon (between noon and 6:00 p.m.)   ℍ II   = 7

Evening (between 6:01 p.m. and 11:59 p.m.)   IIII   = 4

Example 2. A youth counselor wants to inventory the types of questions he asks during house visits and therefore records a conversation he has with a parent. After listening to the recording, he lists all the questions that he posed during the conversation and marks each question as being open or closed:

	Open question	Closed question
Question 1. "Did you write down the agreements together?"		X
Question 2. "Have you reached visitation agreements?"		X
Question 3. "Why not?"	X	

	Open question	Closed question
Question 4. "What are the reasons for the troublesome communication with your ex-husband?"	X	
Question 5. "Does your ex-husband pay the alimony on time?"		X
Question 6. "Why has this situation persisted for so long?"	X	
Totals	3	3

Example 3. A social worker is analyzing the dynamics of a group she is conducting, based on certain activities performed by the members. Her question is, "What behaviors does the client display during the group assignment?"

	Marked	Not marked
Reading	X	
Writing		X
Collaboration	X	

To facilitate interpretation of the data, you can also present results captured in a table in the form of a bar graph.

Nominal and Ordinal Analysis Method 2: Converting Totals to Percentages

The total number of responses can be represented as percentages. By using percentages, the proportional relationship of the answers to each other becomes apparent, and percentages also facilitate comparison of datasets from different groups of participants.

1. Add the total number of answers given by participants.
2. Divide the number of responses for each item by the number in step 1.
3. Round the result up or down.

Example 1. Here are the results of the physical therapist asking what time of day patients prefer to do prescribed exercises but comparing two different service areas:

Which is your preferred time slot for exercising?	Rural area (n = 20)		Urban area (n = 30)	
Night (between midnight and 6:00 a.m.)	6	30%	6	20%
Morning (between 6:01 a.m. and 11:59 a.m.)	3	15%	3	10%
Afternoon (between noon and 6:00 p.m.)	7	35%	9	30%
Evening (between 6:01 p.m. and 11:59 p.m.)	4	20%	12	40%
Totals	20	100%	30	100%

Note: When calculating percentages, it is usual to indicate the total number of participants who are included in the calculation. This is shown as "n =" in the table.

Example 2. A general practitioner is observed by a colleague when speaking with a patient. The consultation is recorded in order to evaluate the doctor's communication skills. The observer writes down the exercise of specific communication skills in five-second intervals. The analysis focuses solely on the frequency of the observed communication skills or actions and not on their duration. The observer did not note if the action actually lasted for five seconds; he only marked its occurrence in those time slots.

	5 sec.	10 sec.	15 sec.	20 sec.	25 sec.	30 sec.	35 sec.
Clarification	X	X				X	X
Asking a question		X	X				
Listening	X			X	X		X

The percentages are then calculated, revealing the most and least observed communication skills.

	Total	Percentage
Clarification	4	40%
Asking a question	2	20%
Listening	4	40%
Total	10	100%

Percentages can be represented easily in graphic formats such as *pie charts*. But also be careful when organizing and interpreting data presented in the form of percentages. One common pitfall is when participants can give multiple responses to a question.

Example. You ask patients to select the nurse or nurses whom they feel have helped them to improve their self-reliance (n = 30):

	Total	Percentage
Nurse 1	15	30%
Nurse 2	22	44%
Nurse 3	13	26%
Total	50	100%

The total of 50 in the table does not indicate the number of participants, but rather that 50 tally marks have been placed on the list. Only 30 patients answered the question (n = 30), but they were allowed to mark more than one response. Concluding that 30 percent of the patients say that Nurse 1 has helped them to improve their self-reliance would be an error. The marked percentage means that 30 percent of the answers relate to the response option "Nurse 1." The table does, however, indicate that Nurse 2 was selected most often and Nurse 3 the least.

This illustrates the importance of indicating the number of participants included in the analysis when presenting the data. This information can be used to analyze the data in a different way, showing instead how often each nurse was selected as a percentage of all responses.

	Selected	Not selected	Total
Nurse 1	15 (50%)	15 (50%)	30 (100%)
Nurse 2	22 (73%)	8 (27%)	30 (100%)
Nurse 3	13 (43%)	17 (57%)	30 (100%)

Knowing that 30 patients answered this particular question allows for a percentage calculation. Fifty percent of the patients in this example feel that Nurse 1 has helped them improve their self-reliance.

Nominal and Ordinal Analysis Method 3: Combining Items

You can combine response options (items) to reduce the data to smaller categories. The new category label needs to cover the content of all the items, and items that do not share many characteristics are better not combined. All response options must be included in the results; none may be omitted.

1. Determine which items can be combined and name the new category.
2. Add the totals of the relevant items.
3. Add the percentages of the relevant items.

Example. Responses to the physical therapist exploring preferred time slots for exercising can be combined into the new categories "a.m." (comprising "night" and "morning") and "p.m." (comprising "afternoon" and "evening").

Which is your preferred time slot for exercising?	Rural area (n = 20)		Urban area (n = 30)	
A.M. (between midnight and 11:59 a.m.)	6 + 3 = 9	45%	6 + 3 = 9	30%
P.M. (between noon and 11:59 p.m.)	7 + 4 = 11	55%	9 + 12 = 21	70%
Total	20	100%	30	100%

Nominal and Ordinal Analysis Method 4: Combining Variables

By combining variables you create new data that may be relevant to the research, and you should consider possible combinations for analysis when you design a research instrument. The tables that display combinations of variables are called *cross tables*. The data in such cross tables can be converted into bar graphs or pie charts.

1. Determine which variables you wish to combine.
2. In the columns, write the names of the items from one variable.
3. In the rows, write the names of items from the other variable.
4. Enter the figures in the appropriate cells based on the collected data.
5. Add the totals for each row and column.
6. Calculate the percentages by cell, column, or row, depending on the information desired.

Example. Our physical therapist asking patients about their preferred time slots for exercising has asked two additional single-response questions:

Where do you live (rural area or urban area)?

What is your gender (male or female?)

She can combine all of her data into the following two tables:

	Rural area (n = 20)		
	Male	Female	Total
Night (between midnight and 6:00 a.m.)	2	4	6
Morning (between 6:01 a.m. and 11:59 a.m.)	3	0	3
Afternoon (between noon and 6:00 p.m.)	4	3	7
Evening (between 6:01 p.m. and 11:59 p.m.)	1	3	4
Total	10	10	20

	Urban area (n = 30)		
	Male	Female	Total
Night (between midnight and 6:00 a.m.)	3	3	6
Morning (between 6:01 a.m. and 11:59 a.m.)	1	2	3
Afternoon (between noon and 6:00 p.m.)	5	4	9
Evening (between 6:00 p.m. and 11:59 p.m.)	4	8	12
Total	13	17	30

Similarly, you can make combinations between interval variables and nominal or ordinal variables.

Example. This table shows a combination of data for two nominal variables ("What is your gender?" and "In which hospital department did you receive your treatment?") and an interval variable ("What is your age?").

Department	Average age Male	Average age Female	Total
Pulmonary	55 (n = 12)	48 (n = 16)	51 (n = 28)
Dermatology	62 (n = 17)	57 (n = 14)	60 (n = 31)
Surgery	63 (n = 13)	64 (n = 15)	64 (n = 28)

Exercise 2. Analyzing Single-Response Questions (see page 202)

Exercise 3. Combining Data (see page 203)

Exercise 4. Analyzing Multiple-Response Questions (see page 203)

Data Analysis for Ordinal Variables in the Form of Rating Scales

Ordinal variables are commonly composed of a rating scale, the respondent selecting from a range of options representing a gradation. The range of the scale is equal to the number of options. For instance, you can view a question with a three-choice rating scale as a single-response question with three response options. You can use nominal and ordinal analysis methods 1–3 for this purpose and method 4 when you combine a rating scale question with another type of single-response question, for example, when calculating the difference in responses between boys and girls to the same rating scale question.

Most researchers assume that participants consider the value differences between the items of a rating scale to be equal, which is why the items on these scales may be replaced by numbers with equal-value intervals (a five-item scale becomes a numbered scale with a range of 1–5, and a seven-item scale becomes a numbered scale with a range of 1–7). With this format, the scales render numbered results. The following example shows that the participant selected the fourth item:

Completely agree ←OOO●O→ Completely disagree (value = 4)

When you convert a scale to numbers, you can perform calculations with the data. For example, if the average score on a five-point scale is 3.4, it means that the group average is between the third and fourth item. Converting a rating scale to numbers also enables you to apply interval analysis methods 1–4.

Data Analysis for Standardized Tests

Standardized tests—regarding, for example, life satisfaction (e.g., Satisfaction with Life Scale, or SWL), depression (e.g., PHQ-9 Depression Test), or activities of daily living (e.g., Instrumental Activities of Daily Living Scale, or IADL)—are commonly used in practitioner research. There are several advantages: (1) the instruments for data collection are ready to use, (2) the instruments have been shown to be valid in various practice settings, and (3) the results of your study can be compared with the work of other practitioner researchers using the same instrument. Each test has its own procedure for collecting and analyzing the data, which you should follow carefully. Several tests yield a numerical score that you can treat as an interval variable, applying the appropriate methods as described throughout this section.

6.3. Analyzing Qualitative Data

Nonnumerical research data can take various forms, such as text (answers to open questions, fragments from literature, open-observation reports), video and/or audio recordings, pictures, chart notes, or detailed mind maps. This type of data is less structured and thus cannot be transformed into numbers, which makes the analysis process more complex. Therefore, you need to take steps to add structure to the data, making it amenable to analysis.

Included here are several basic methods to analyze qualitative data in the form of text. Analysis of audio and video data is also discussed, followed by analysis of results from open tests.

Data Analysis for Texts

Open-ended questions do not have predetermined response options. The resulting data can, therefore, vary greatly between participants, taking on many forms or directions. Your research question will help you determine which of the following methods of analysis is the most suitable for your study.

Text Analysis Method 1: Labeling and Categorizing Noteworthy Text Fragments

The process of collecting qualitative data generally yields high volumes of text. A 10-minute conversation can easily result in a three-page transcript. You can divide text data into parts based on relevance and/or significance, which involves, for instance, grouping fragments—a few words, lines, or statements related to the same topic. You subsequently assign these fragments a category label in a process called *coding*. In open coding, you do not create categories before you start the analysis; the categories are formed during the process of analysis and are based on the research data. The categories stand for the underlying themes or opinions found in the fragments. This is called an *inductive* process, and it is best suited for situations where the research is exploratory in nature, not assuming in advance certain categories for the analysis. The list of categories that you create constitutes the primary result of the data analysis.

> *Example.* You are interested in the way that the counselors in a residential group for children with behavioral problems address the children's feelings of homesickness. A committee of parents and guardians indicates that no official guidelines regarding this subject have been issued, and a joint decision is reached that you will inventory the current practices and approaches of the group counselors regarding homesickness. You organize a group interview with several of the counselors and write a report about your findings. You divide this report into noteworthy fragments. In ad-

dition, you come up with a category label for each fragment regarding the approaches that the group counselors use to address homesickness.

Text fragment 1: "I just had a long talk with M. about his family yesterday. It's something I always do when I see that kids are sad."
   Category label: dialogue

Text fragment 2: "I try to organize fun activities for children who are feeling homesick to make them forget their distress. They are completely absorbed by activities like football, movies, or computer games."
   Category label: distraction

Text fragment 3: "I don't think there are many children in my group that are homesick, really. If they are sad, it is usually because of a conflict within the group and I try to talk to the child about the issue. This often relieves the sadness."
   Category label: considering other causes

Text fragment 4: "I don't think homesickness is the most important issue right now. Yesterday, one of the children mentioned that the taxi is always too late to pick them up."
   This fragment is not relevant and will be excluded.

Text fragment 5: "The first thing I do is find a quiet spot to talk with the children."
   Category label: dialogue

Text fragment 6: "I then look for ways to ease the pain, like allowing a phone call to their parents."
   Category label: facilitating contact with family or guardians

Text fragment 7: "Or we go through the family album together."
   Category label: looking at photographs

Text Analysis Method 2: Analyzing Data Based on Predetermined Categories

Contrary to the inductive coding method, where categories are created during the data analysis, here you create the categories using a *deductive* method. This means that you set the relevant categories before commencing the data analysis. The categories are based on the insight that you gained from the literature review and from professional practice. You match text fragments that are relevant to the research question to the listed categories. You have likely already used these categories when designing your research instruments.

1. Write down the question that the data analysis needs to answer.

2. Create categories to analyze the information based on the literature review and the research instruments used for data collection.

3. Divide the collected data (such as observation and interview reports) into smaller, noteworthy fragments (see text analysis method 1).

4. For each separate category, mark relevant passages in the text. You may have to create new categories for fragments that do not fit into any of the existing categories.

Example. Residential counselors indicate that the results from the annual quantitative resident satisfaction survey are not useful unless more background information accompanies the answers. In hopes of gaining more insight, the organization supplements the annual survey with qualitative interviews and an observation study with 12 residents regarding the everyday conditions in the home. These residents were selected prior to starting the research project and have agreed to participate. They are observed intensely by several of the residential counselors during joint activities.

The observers also note any significant events that occur during the period that they shadow the residents. Individual interviews are also conducted. The observation protocol and the interview guide are based on a literature review of resident satisfaction. These categories are the layout of the residents' rooms, resident-counselor interaction, social contacts with other residents, the activities program, and the quality of the food, among others. The same categories are used to structure the analysis of the observation and interview reports, as well as the counselors' notes.

You can perform different analyses once the relevant data has been organized into categories. For example, you can tally the number of responses fitting into a particular category (frequency), establish the sequence or combination of particular categories, or compare the frequency of categories for two or more groups (such as boys and girls). This step can result in a numerical analysis of the data.

Example: You ask youth workers to describe their own professional qualities. You then divide these descriptions into noteworthy text fragments, with each fragment describing one single quality. You base the categories you use on the professional competencies of youth workers found on the Act for Youth website (http://actforyouth.net), and as outlined in your literature review, and file each fragment into the appropriate category. You subsequently tally how often the youth workers have indicated that a particular competency is one of their strong points. This calculation shows that the highest scoring competency is "curriculum (program activities)."

Text Analysis Method 3: Thematic Coding

Similar to the previous method, thematic analysis uses previously determined central themes. However, contrary to it, your focus is less on the frequency of these themes but rather on the manner in which the themes emerge from the text as well as their interrelationship (connections and deeper meaning). In such an analysis, you often first present a motto that represents the idea of a respondent or author of a text source. This can be a short quotation or a short characterization. You then concisely summarize the conversation or the text source. The summary depicts the reasoning and experience of the participant or source, thus providing more background and the "story" behind the data. You can add this summary to the motto. If you reduce each data source to its most essential elements in this way, it is possible to compare it with other data sources (for example, by using horizontal comparison, which is the method to be discussed). Comparing the mottos and summaries of different respondents or sources allows you to go deeper into interrelationships, explanations, and patterns than is possible using text analysis methods 1 and 2.

Example. In recent years, a nursing home has seen a large influx of new health care professionals. Leo wishes to find out how his colleagues felt about their onboarding experience so he can use the results to develop a coaching track for future nurses who start working at the facility. He speaks extensively with six nurses on an individual basis. He decides to code the reports of these discussions thematically. He has selected several key themes that are relevant to early-career nurses in the nursing home. One of the themes is labeled "support of colleagues." From each of the six interview reports, he chooses a quotation (a motto) that is typical of how the nurse feels about this theme. He then adds a summary of each conversation.

Motto: "Colleagues were willing to answer my questions but took hardly any initiative to ask me questions or to explain."

Summary: *A year and a half ago L. came to work at this location. Before that, she worked at a different nursing home. At this previous location she acted as a team leader, although this was not her formal position. She commented that she had to get used to this new department at the start, because her role here was clearly different. Occasionally this led to minor conflicts with her colleagues. As a result, it made her feel like she was sometimes isolated, and she was not very comfortable in her new working environment. If she had any questions, her colleagues were usually willing to answer them. She talked a lot with colleagues about procedures and their daily routines. To her, it seemed that her colleagues were often very busy. They asked her few questions and seemed to assume that she would be all right.*

After analyzing all six reports this way, Leo draws parallels between his findings. The comparisons help him to get a better idea about workplace interactions and available nursing staff support.

Text Analysis Method 4: Horizontal Comparison

Horizontal comparison enables you to evaluate the answers of different individuals to the same open question. You juxtapose all the answers, mark any significant parallels or differences, and subsequently compose a brief synopsis of the findings. In essence, you summarize the various answers and then compare them. Horizontal comparison is only feasible with a limited number of data sources. The steps are as follows:

1. Create an analysis table.
2. In the first column, note the research question for which the data will be compared horizontally. Indicate your purpose for the comparison.
3. The following columns contain the data from each source. Create one column for each source, entering only relevant content. Reserve the last column for conclusions.

4. Review the data for each source and mark the parts that contribute to answering the research question.

5. Formulate general conclusions based on the marked fragments, discussing both similarities and differences.

Example. Your practice has rearranged its office space so as to be more patient-friendly. You have interviewed three patients about your practice's new layout in a semi-structured interview. Using horizontal comparison, you have compared their responses and come to some conclusions for next steps.

	Answer Patient 1	Answer Patient 2	Answer Patient 3	Conclusions
Question 1: How do you like the new layout of the work area? *Motive:* I want to find out if the patients are happy with the new layout of the work area and/or if they think improvements can be made.	I'm <u>very happy with the new lay-out.</u> I did not expect it to be <u>so nice.</u> I do <u>miss having my own locker.</u>	It <u>took some getting used to,</u> but I realize now that I <u>actually like the</u> new layout. I like being able to <u>work with others</u> now.	I <u>am satisfied,</u> but kind of <u>miss the old layout.</u> I notice that the <u>new layout promotes interaction.</u> Maybe the <u>room can be split,</u> so that there is a <u>space to work individually</u> as well.	The three patients are mostly happy. A few improvements have been suggested: quiet, more secluded areas to work individually, and personal storage space.

Question 2: . . .

Motive: . . .

Text Analysis Method 5: Illustrating Data Analysis Results

To highlight the story behind the data, you can supplement the results of the data analysis with concrete examples or brief text fragments:

Example. You would like to know what parents and guardians think about the atmosphere in the residential group for patients with a mental disability. You distribute a short questionnaire containing several statements, one of which is: "My son/daughter likes the range of group activities in the residential group." The respondents can indicate whether they agree or disagree and have the option to elaborate in the comments box. Several of the respondents provide feedback. For example:

"Julia loved the Christmas dinner."

"Mia perks up when we ask about the activities in the group. She often speaks about designing the seasonal table, the creative assignments, and decorating the common room for birthdays."

"The many activities you organize are a boon for most residents. Our Jerry cannot handle too well the commotion and tension that are sometimes associated with these activities. He cannot put this into words as such, but we do notice it in his behavior."

"We can see that Jeannie really enjoys the group activities. Personally, we feel there could be more focus on sports and exercise."

The analysis shows that the majority of the parents agree with the statement. In the report, you include (anonymous) comments and suggestions from respondents to illustrate both affirmative and negative answers. The names used should not be the real names of the participants or their family members.

Exercise 5. Qualitative Content Analysis (see page 204)

Exercise 6. Dividing Text into Noteworthy Parts (see page 204)

Data Analysis for Audio or Visual Data

Audio and video materials yield a substantial amount of data, as mentioned before. You can analyze video data by watching the footage and documenting the findings in an observation or comparison chart. For audio material, the recommended method involves first transcribing the recording and subsequently analyzing the text. As described earlier, the resulting coding can be quantitative or qualitative in form. For quantitative data, use nominal and ordinal analysis methods 1–4; for qualitative data, use text analysis methods 1–5.

You may have asked participants to create visual representations of their answers, such as drawings or schematic depictions (such as mind maps or concepts maps). Such material is often difficult to interpret without further explanation from the participants. You can ask the creator of a drawing for clarification if you are going to include it in the analysis. For each drawing, write a report on the participant's explanation of the descriptions and labels. You can analyze these reports using text analysis methods 1–5. You can always use the drawings in their original format to illustrate your research results (text analysis method 5).

> *Example.* You ask local senior citizens to draw their ideal meeting area. You can review and describe these sketches based on several parameters, such as location, furniture arrangement, and use of color. The parameters are based on your research question, and you can horizontally compare the descriptions of the drawings and other creative input (text analysis method 4). You can also ask the creators of the pieces for background on their work. You analyze these extra details and put them to paper using text analysis methods 1–5.

Data Analysis for Testing Using Open-Ended Questions

Testing does not need to be done using standardized, quantitative instruments. You can also test certain qualities of participants (e.g., level of knowledge or success in treatment) by asking open-ended questions that you formulate yourself. You formulate the categories for the quality you are testing in advance and then analyze the answers to the questions according to these categories. The aim is to file the participants' answers under the corresponding categories (e.g., learning objectives or goals for treatment), either per individual or per group. You can use text analysis methods 1–5 to accomplish this.

Example. A Health Department health educator organizes safer-sex education projects at high schools. She asks the students to write a report on the subject at the end of the project to demonstrate what they have learned. The students are required to explore several set topics. The health educator analyzes the reports based on the educational objectives. She divides the students' reports into note-worthy passages and files these under the educational objectives but does so only for those text fragments that demonstrate the students' comprehension of the topic. After she analyzes all the reports, the health educator finds that two of the required topics remain blank. This could indicate that the project did not help the students to achieve those particular educational objectives. Based on this in-formation, the health educator could decide to modify the content of the project and increase the focus on these less-understood topics. Alternatively, she could first find out why the students did not comment on these subjects, as there could be several possible reasons for the omissions.

6.4. Forming Conclusions

Once your analysis has yielded results, you can start forming conclusions (figure 6.3). In this systematic process, you formulate short and concise answers to the main research question and its corresponding sub-questions. These answers are supposed to provide you with more insight into the practice problem and to a possible solution.

The conclusions should logically flow from the collected data. It is therefore best to create a table that indicates which questions you are answering, what your conclusions are, and on which analysis results you base these conclusions.

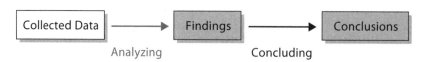

Figure 6.3

The conclusion process turns findings into research conclusions

Example. You are wanting to improve an after-school youth program based on the feedback of the users and potential users of the program. You make two conclu-sions based on your research.

Research sub-question: What should be the focus of the after-school program in the youth center from the perspective of local youth?

Conclusion 1: The after-school program should focus primarily on sports, dance, computers, and music.	*Reference*: See summary table 3 for the analysis results of the answers to questions 4 and 5 of the questionnaire. These topics of interest score 50% or higher.
Conclusion 2: The after-school program should be categorically different than the regular curriculum in school, with more room for the children's own preferences.	*Reference*: See summary table 4 for the most important findings of the group interviews with the children. This detail was mentioned in three of the four group interviews.

Phrase the conclusions in clear and unambiguous terms to ensure that each reader interprets them the same way, though this objective is never 100 percent attainable as people have different assumptions and opinions. It is important that you test your conclusions against the results of the analysis. Beware of drawing more precise conclusions than the analysis results allow for or of letting personal opinions pervade the text. If you draw conclusions that are not based on the analysis results, these statements cannot be called conclusions. You can include your personal opinion in a separate discussion section of the research report, where you can also state predictions on the outlook for the future, related questions, points of contention, and new thoughts resulting from the research. Structuring your research report this way separates your findings from your personal ideas and advice (see chapter 8).

Step-by-Step Guide for Drawing Conclusions

The following guide can help you to form conclusions, and the example scenario walks through steps 1–5.

1. Sort the analysis results per sub-question (if this has not been done yet).

2. Review the analysis results for each sub-question. Based on these results, formulate short statements in answer to the individual questions.

3. Rephrase the answers clearly and unambiguously, and link the answers to the research context. This way, readers can comprehend the results that you present in your research report.

4. Illustrate the conclusions with fragments from the collected data, if necessary.

5. Clearly make record in a table of each sub-question you're answering, what conclusions you draw, and on which analysis results these conclusions are based.

6. Draw parallels between the answers to the sub-questions and, if possible, answer the main research question. The main question can occasionally be answered by referring to answers to sub-questions.

7. Ask other people to read both your conclusions and the results of the analysis in order to verify the accuracy of the conclusions that you formed.

Example Scenario: Steps 1–5 of Drawing a Research Conclusion

A head nurse researches the extent to which the organization's policies have led to observable changes in the practices and/or actions of the nurses in the urology department. He sorts the analysis results for the following two sub-questions (steps 1–2):

Sub-question 1. How are the policies divided over the eight themes in the organization's policy manual?

- One-third of the policies in the manual imply changes that directly impact the patients in the hospital.
- No policies were formulated to increase staff input in the decision-making process.

Sub-question 2. To what degree did nursing staff change their practices after the implementation of the policy "Do not discuss sensitive patient information during visiting hours"?

- The policy has not led to observable changes in the nurses' actions, according to 28 out of 30 respondents.

The statement "The policy strategies have not led to observable change in nurses' actions, according to 28 out of 30 respondents" is rephrased (step 3) to become the following conclusion:

"Virtually the entire urology nursing staff (93 percent) indicate that the policy statement 'Do not discuss sensitive patient information during visiting hours' did not lead to visible changes in the practices of the nursing staff in the department."

One of the nurses made the following comment during a group interview: "Colleagues still discuss patients' situations in the presence of family members, friends, and/or acquaintances. The policy clearly states that the privacy of the patient is paramount and needs to be respected during visiting hours." The head nurse adds this statement to the aforementioned conclusion (step 4) and documents it in the conclusions table (step 5).

Sub-question: To what degree did nursing staff change their practices after the implementation of the policy "Do not discuss sensitive patient information during visiting hours"?

Conclusion 1: Virtually the entire urology nursing staff (93 percent) indicate that the policy statement "Do not discuss sensitive patient information during visiting hours" did not lead to visible changes in the practices of the nursing staff in the department.	*Reference*: See summary table 3 with the analysis results of question 4 of the questionnaire.
As one person stated during the interviews, "Colleagues still discuss patients' situations in the presence of family members, friends, and/or acquaintances. The policy clearly states that the privacy of the patient is paramount and needs to be respected during visiting hours."	

Use Common Sense

Continually run mental checks on the logic and validity of your conclusions and remain critical with regards to the results of your research.

> *Example.* You plan to distribute a survey among therapists to assess their sense of security in the workplace. If the therapists receive these questions immediately after a serious incident took place, the resulting answers will likely vary greatly from responses to a survey held during an uneventful period. The data collected just after the incident would likely lead to the conclusion that the sense of security is very low. The question then becomes if this is, in fact, a reasonable conclusion.

Use Digital Tools

You can simplify data analysis with many digital tools and online resources, such as word processing programs for analyzing text fragments or creating and analyzing graphic data (e.g., images, mind maps, or concept maps). Qualitative data is sometimes analyzed with qualitative analysis software, such as Atlas.ti or MAXQDA. Statistics can be calculated in spreadsheet software such as Microsoft Excel or Calc, or in specific statistical analysis software such as SPSS or GNU PSPP. These tools can greatly reduce the time required to achieve results.

Document Your Steps Accurately

Properly document collected data as well as any findings from the analysis of the results. The documentation shows other interested parties how you reached your conclusions, and it enables you to reuse the data in future research.

> *Example.* Six months earlier, you asked the children in the after-school care center where you work how they like the fine-motor-skills toys at the center. Follow-up discussions indicated that the children like some toys less than others because they are not as familiar with them. You therefore decided to actively encourage the children to play with these less-familiar toys so they can get comfortable using them. Six months later, you wish to revisit the issue, but realize that there is little information that was recorded from that experience. You found a synopsis of the findings, but you no longer have the original data nor can you remember the method of analysis. This complicates a comparison between the two datasets.

Rely on Other People

Involve your participants in reflecting on instrument questions before they are asked (i.e., pretest the instrument) and to verify the findings by getting feedback from them after their participation, for instance, by asking participants to review the summary of an interview to see if they agree. You can increase the validity and reliability of the research by asking others to review the analysis.

> *Example.* Almost all the nurses in a perinatal clinic disagree with the following questionnaire statement: "I always take great pleasure in providing care to patients." You are inclined to assume the nurses do not enjoy their work very much, but to confirm this you consult several of the staff. These conversations show that most of the nurses do, in fact, enjoy their work, but that they gave a negative answer because the statement included the word "always." You decide to remove "always" from the statement and readminister the questionnaire later. It is likely the reactions to this particular statement will be more positive.

Feedback on the data from multiple stakeholders with varying perspectives prevents you from systematically influencing the analysis process due to conscious or unconscious bias.

> *Example.* Several therapists are interviewed about the differences between cognitive behavioral therapy and gestalt therapy for patients with postnatal (postpartum) depression. However, the interview reports are analyzed by a single therapist. If that therapist fervently supports cognitive behavioral therapy, he may very well unconsciously reach different conclusions than a therapist who prefers Gestalt therapy. Therefore, it would be preferable to have multiple individuals analyze this data.

Only Examine or Measure What You Need to Know

During the analysis and conclusion phase, you may find that the methods of data collection and the research instruments you used did not gather the information you needed to answer the research question. In this case, you will have to repeat (all or part of) the data collection process in a different manner.

> *Example 1.* As leader of a multidisciplinary team, you wish to know what cooperation skills your colleagues display when working on a case scenario during a two-day communication training. The observation charts you prepared lack several parameters related to task allocation between members of the group. During the observation you therefore miss behavior or actions that may be important in regard to your research question.

Example 2. You wish to draw up individual movement therapy plans for all your patients. To correctly estimate the patients' individual level of motor function, you ask each patient to perform several exercises. However, the exercises are too simple for everyone in the group, and there is a lack of differentiation of exercises by ability. As a result, you do not gain further insight into the patients' individual motor skills.

Example 3. To find out what information patients miss on the organization's website, you design an online questionnaire with rating questions. The questionnaire is automatically opened when online visitors view the site. As access to the website is not restricted, the questionnaire is not only presented to patients but to every other visitor to the site as well. When you perform the data analysis, it proves impossible to determine which answers were submitted by patients and which ones by other respondents.

Take Data Dispersion (Sufficiently) into Account

Using averages to give a summary of the collected data is a common practice, but the reality may not always correspond to the calculated average.

Example. The director of a mental health institution values continuing education on new treatment methods and organizes a meeting to introduce a recently developed method. At the end of the meeting, the director asks the assembled counselors to rate on a scale of 1–7 the option of permanently incorporating this new method into the standard procedures. The two extreme values indicate "This treatment should not become part of the treatment program" and "The method should become a fixed part of the treatment program." Ten of the 30 counselors are so positive that they rate the suggested introduction a 7 out of 7. The other staff members are more cautious: six counselors mark a score of 2, and 14 counselors rate the idea with a score of 3. These scores indicate that the majority of staff members prefer not to make the treatment a fixture in the institution's standard procedures.

The director adds all the scores and divides the total by the number of participating counselors, which generally is a valid calculation for this type of question. The average score is 4.13 (out of 7) and the director therefore concludes that the new method should be included permanently in the program.

A closer look at the scores would have told the director that the majority of the 30 counselors gave the new method a score of 3 or less. The higher average is due to the 10 counselors that gave the maximum score.

This example illustrates the importance of considering score dispersion. A good measure for this is the standard deviation. A large standard deviation means a significant difference in the scores and is often a reason to review the data in the form of a table, bar chart, or line graph. In some cases, the median may be a better representation of the data than the average (see section 6.2).

Losing Sight of Background Information

Numbers are a helpful way of summarizing the collected data, but they only represent part of the reality. Keep a critical view and link your results to other available data as well as the relevant research context. Be cautious when generalizing conclusions.

Example 1. An addiction counselor wants to measure the influence that the topic of dialogue has on patient interaction during group sessions, so he captures two meetings on video. The first session is based on the patients' personal experiences, while the second session uses fictional cases as the subject for discussion. The counselor watches the footage and notes patient interactions. After analyzing the data from both sessions, he notices that less interaction occurred during the first session. He therefore concludes that the second form of dialogue is more effective in stimulating patient interaction.

While the counselor's conclusion may be correct, it is not well founded. Less visible interaction during the first session may have also been the result of the presence of a video camera—an unfamiliar situation for the patients. Another reason could be that patients needed to get used to this new group. Performing several more observations would have added weight to the counselor's conclusions.

Example 2. You have captured the following data about the level of education of nursing-home staff as it relates to their gender.

	Male	Female
High school	40% (n = 2)	20% (n = 1)
College	60% (n = 3)	60% (n = 3)
Graduate	0% (n = 0)	20% (n = 1)
Total	100% (n = 5)	100% (n = 5)

These percentages could lead to the following conclusions:

- 40 percent of male staff and 20 percent of female staff have a high-school level education.
- Only female staff members have graduate degrees.

The most important question here is whether 10 staff members are really representative of the entire staff. To really gain insight into the different levels of education, more staff members need to be surveyed.

Limited numbers do not mean that you cannot draw any conclusions at all, but the conclusions reached for small groups usually cannot be generalized to a larger population (in this case, the entire staff of the nursing home). It is important to note that small changes in limited groups can lead to large changes in the outcome of the research. You must mention this problem when reporting and presenting the research results for small sample sizes.

Avoid Flawed Reasoning

One error in data analysis that is frequently made is reverse reasoning.

Example. Suppose 25 percent of male colleagues come to work reluctantly. Your conclusion therefore is 75 percent of male colleagues come to work eagerly.

This is hardly a valid conclusion, as the participants were not asked if they go to work eagerly. You can only realistically conclude that 75 percent do not go to work reluctantly.

Take Missing or Incorrect Data into Account

Data collection is not always complete, due to, for instance, interrupted observations, blank answers on questionnaires, or group discussions that run out of time. Occasionally, respondents may mark several responses where you actually only allow a single one.

Example. You survey 30 clients in a medical debt restructuring program as to how they spend their income. One of the questions relates to contractual financial obligations that the clients have entered into during the past year. Only one of the clients answers this question. It could be that the other clients did not understand the question. The client that did answer the question indicates that he did not sign any contracts with financial obligations. You therefore conclude that, in general, the clients did not enter into any contractual financial obligations.

The survey in this example suffers from *nonresponse* (answers left blank by respondents), which you must consider when forming your conclusions. No answers mean no data on which to base conclusions. The implication here could be that you cannot form a valid conclusion about this question due to a lack of data. You need to consider instances of nonresponse carefully. If insufficient data is returned to draw conclusions from, you will have to collect new data. Other reasons to collect new data can be that the number of respondents is too limited, that there was an insufficient number of relevant answers, or that the method of data collection was too one-sided (i.e., insufficient triangulation; see section 1.4). Having contingencies on hand is good practice in case the research activities that you intended to base your conclusions on do not yield sufficient data.

Use common sense for these decisions, and always elaborate on the actions taken with regards to missing or inadequate data when presenting your research results.

Exercise 7. Linking Analysis Results to Conclusions (see page 205)

Exercise 8. Establishing the Validity of Conclusions (see page 205)

6.6. Summary

This chapter described the steps for analyzing data to form conclusions:

1. Sorting the collected data per sub-question
2. Reducing, combining, and/or transforming the collected data
3. Presenting the analysis results (findings)
4. Forming clear and sound conclusions based on the findings

Two forms of data are distinguished: quantitative and qualitative. Analysis of the latter is more labor-intensive and time-consuming, as you need to structure the data before you can launch the process of analysis. This is not the case for quantitative data. You can use several methods of analysis for both types of data, and you must always keep the research question in mind during data analysis.

The conclusions that you form must answer the research question. The conclusions that you report must be logical for the reader in the context of the data you collected.

Important points to consider during the analysis and conclusion process are (1) use common sense, (2) use digital tools when possible, (3) maintain solid documentation, (4) use appropriate instruments, (5) take data dispersion into account, (6) keep background information and context in mind, (7) be cautious when generalizing conclusions, (8) avoid reverse reasoning, and (9) take missing data into account. Further, you can increase the validity and reliability of the research by asking others to review the analysis.

EXERCISES

Exercise 1. Asking Questions with Interval Variables

Survey question: How many friends do you have in the after-school program?

Answers by 10 children in group A: 3, 5, 1, 7, 4, 5, 34, 6, 2, 2

Answers by 10 children in group B: 2, 5, 7, 6, 5, 1, 4, 3, 3, 1

Questions and assignments:

1. Calculate the average number of friends for the children in both groups.
2. Find the median of the number of friends for the children in both groups.
3. Do you think the data is best represented by the average or the median?
4. Which conclusion(s) can you form based on the data?

Exercise 2. Analyzing Single-Response Questions

Survey question: A therapy session of 25 minutes is sufficiently long.

o True (selected 41 times)

o False (selected 62 times)

(n = 103)

Questions and assignments:

    1. What does "n = 103" mean?

    2. Have all respondents answered the question?

    3. Convert the totals to percentages.

Exercise 3. Combining Data

Research question 1: What is your gender? (1 = male, 2 = female)

Research question 2: What is the highest degree or level of education that you have completed? (1 = high school, 2 = college, 3 = graduate school)

Data table:

Respondent (R)	Question 1	Question 2
R1	1	1
R2	1	2
R3	2	1
R4	2	1
R5	1	3
R6	2	3
R7	1	2
R8	2	1
R9	1	3
R10	1	1

Questions and assignments:

    1. How many respondents answered the questions?

    2. Combine the answers to question 1 with the answers to question 2 in a new table.

    3. Convert the totals to percentages.

    4. What conclusion(s) can you form based on this data?

Exercise 4. Analyzing Multiple-Response Questions

On a weekly basis, I communicate with patients (check all that apply):

    ☐ by phone (selected 63 times)

    ☐ by email (selected 82 times)

    ☐ by social media (selected 12 times)

    ☐ at their home (selected 26 times)

    ☐ at the clinic (selected 42 times)

      (n = 90)

Questions and assignment:

1. How many boxes did each respondent tick on average?
2. Convert the totals to percentages.
3. What conclusion(s) can you form based on this data?

Exercise 5. Qualitative Content Analysis

Perform this exercise in a group. Start by jointly formulating one open interview question to discuss. Examples of such questions are:

Which factors are essential for treatments to be successful?

What are your experiences with the new guidelines?

What is the best format for the organization's meetings, in your opinion?

After you've agreed on a question, conduct short discussions among members of the group and write a brief report of answers given to the question. Make copies of the report and distribute these within the entire group.

Analyze the report using one of the methods for analyzing qualitative data and formulate a conclusion to the interview question. If this action is performed by each group member individually, the results can be compared afterward in the group.

Exercise 6. Dividing Text into Noteworthy Parts

Review the following observation report on three clients with mental disabilities made during their workday in a gift shop by a social worker. Working in the shop is part of a new day-activity program of the organization that is being developed and tested by staff members. The social worker hopes that this setting will provide insight into the question, "How do clients handle shop customers' questions?"

Divide the observation report into meaningful fragments, omitting irrelevant text. Label the noteworthy fragments.

Location: Gift shop
Date: December 10, 2020
Time: 11:30 a.m.–12:30 p.m.

J paces in front of the shop door. He keeps checking his watch and asks (supervisor) L if he can open the shop. L says that it is almost time and that he can officially open the shop. C and A are inside, rearranging items here and there.

As the first customer enters the shop, J and A immediately approach him and almost simultaneously ask him if he wants to buy something. The customer says maybe, but that he would first like to look around. J lists all the items in the shop to the customer. A corrects J because he mentions an item that is not for sale in the shop (a fruit basket).

The customer browses a short time, followed closely by J and A. The customer asks C, who is standing in a corner of the shop, if he has any gift ideas for a newborn. C reacts by handing the customer a stuffed panda and asking him if he wants it wrapped. The client says he would like to know the price first. J and A call out different prices, while C does not react to the customer's question. The customer asks C again how much the panda costs. C walks over to the supervisor and asks her if she knows how much it costs. The supervisor whispers the price ($6) in C's ear, and he tells the customer this. The customer says he would like to buy the panda and have it wrapped. That same instant, two other customers enter the shop.

J approaches the two new customers and tells them they will have to wait as another customer is being attended to. The two customers stand in the doorway. The supervisor indicates that they can come in and look around. J reacts to the supervisor's action by nodding to the customers and saying it's ok to look around. A helps C to wrap the stuffed panda that the first customer bought. The two new customers are together and want to know if gifts can be exchanged. J shakes his head and says that exchanging gifts is impossible. The supervisor calls J over and explains what the customers mean by "exchanging." J then walks back to the customers and says exchanges are possible. A calls out from behind the cash register that they do have to show a receipt, otherwise exchanging gifts really is impossible. . . .

Exercise 7. Linking Analysis Results to Conclusions

List the analysis results that could lead to the following conclusions. Describe the required research activities as concretely as possible.

1. The patients in a residential group need at least 30 minutes of exercise daily.
2. The new safe-internet project is aimed at actively educating youth about the possibilities and the dangers of the internet.
3. Both therapists and management are very satisfied with the new patient registration system. The therapists think that the system should be modified to also store video recordings and images.
4. Meetings should be held more often, but they should be shorter in duration.
5. Scheduling appointments outside of office hours with the physical therapist should be possible.
6. Virtually all clients indicate that they are no longer dependent on the job coach after going to work five days a week for three months.
7. Longer consultations lead to higher patient satisfaction in the dental clinic.

Exercise 8. Establishing the Validity of Conclusions

Consider the following conclusions, either individually or in a group. Why are these conclusions not sound?

1. The patients in the morning group are better than the ones in the afternoon group.
2. I don't think that the new layout of the department is in line with the vision of proper care.

3. Different requirements need to be put in place for hiring new colleagues.

4. The therapists think it is unwise to deny patients a say in deciding the duration and content of their treatment.

5. Broadening the scope of both health care and social work may lead to more competition between providers.

7 | Design and Innovation

ractitioner research always starts with an orientation and problem analysis. If this reveals that existing practices need to be improved, you may decide to systematically design and test an intervention to create a solution to your practice problem.

In section 7.1, we introduce design research, followed by different types of interventions in section 7.2. In section 7.3, we describe the steps taken in the first phase of design research, focusing on the design principles. A similar procedure is used during the second phase—the Innovation Loop (figure 7.1)—that is described in section 7.4. Lastly, the rapid prototyping design method is presented in section 7.5, followed by a brief summary of the chapter and relevant exercises.

7.1. An Introduction to Design Research

All practitioner research projects aim to improve practice by providing new insights for solving a specific practice problem. Sometimes the best solution to a problem is developing and testing a new intervention. Following the steps of the Innovation Loop enables you to do that.

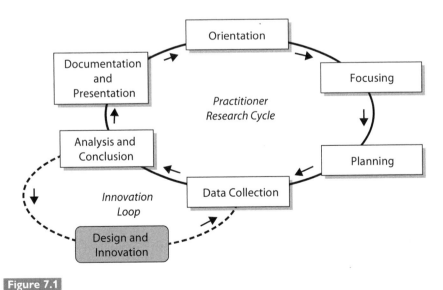

Figure 7.1

Key components of practitioner research: Design and Innovation

Examples of interventions you may want to design are new treatment methods, worksheets for clients/patients, manuals for colleagues, educational programs, triage procedures, changes to the layout of a particular space, patient-provider interaction protocols, informational leaflets or websites, or patient intake checklists. Any new intervention intended to improve practice is an *innovation*. Van Leeuwen (2004) writes that an innovation is an idea, custom, or object that the target group, such as an individual user or an organization, perceives as novel. It is irrelevant whether the idea is, in fact, new; it is the user's perception of novelty that matters. Innovation, therefore, is not so much about inventing as it is about reinventing existing solutions.

The process of designing an innovation is complex and requires more than just having a good idea. The main challenge is finding a solution to the practice problem that works in everyday practice and is supported by your colleagues, clients/patients, and other stakeholders.

> *Example.* A home care organization develops a website to facilitate communication with elderly patients. The team that proposes the idea aspires to make it simple for patients to contact home care professionals at any time through the site. When the intervention is put into practice, it becomes obvious that the limited computer skills and slow internet connections of many of the patients were not taken into account. Additionally, many staff members prefer more direct contact (visit or telephone) over the electronic medium.

It is important to involve those who will use or be affected by your intervention, such as management, colleagues, and clients/patients. They can provide valuable feedback during both the design and testing process.

Design research consists of two phases: diagnosis of the practice problem and designing a solution (Andriessen, 2011). Diagnosis of the practice problem consists of *exploratory research*, where you investigate the problem by collecting data and analyze the data to identify key elements for a possible solution to the practice problem. In this book, these elements are called *design principles*.

The second phase (designing a solution) is what we have named the *Innovation Loop*. The loop guides the development and implementation of the intervention:

1. The intervention is designed, based on the design principles formulated in phase 1.

2. The intervention is implemented in a test phase, and data is collected and analyzed during the process.

3. If the data collected during the test phase shows that the intervention is incomplete, does not meet the design principles, or does not achieve the intended goal (i.e., solution of the practice problem), then changes in the design are necessary.

4. The cycle of designing, testing, collecting data, analyzing, and improving is repeated until the intervention meets the design principles and provides a solution to the practice problem.

Example. The staff of a treatment program for adolescents with diagnoses on the autism spectrum notice that conflict frequently arises about the program rules. A problem analysis shows that a substantial part of the problem stems from the differences between the rules at home and those in the program. The providers decide to focus on this difference and look for a possible solution. They speak to the adolescents and their families, visit other programs, and review journal articles. Based on the information they gather, a set of design principles is formulated that aim for greater involvement of parents/guardians and other informal caregivers so as to harmonize the program rules with the home environment, thus providing more consistency in the support provided to the adolescents.

The team subsequently designs an intervention based on the design principles. One of the intervention components is the creation of a committee composed of adolescents, family members, and providers. The committee convenes monthly to discuss the positive and negative experiences during daily activities at home and in the program. The intervention is tested for six months and proves to be unsuccessful in reducing conflict. Several family members attend sporadically, finding it difficult to meet in the afternoon. Many committee members doubt the usefulness of participating in the monthly meetings, saying they are too infrequent. Modifications are made; the meetings are conducted biweekly in the evening. Attendance of the meetings on the part of family members improves and the exchange at the meetings becomes more focused. The result is a reduction of conflict, both at home and in the program.

This example illustrates that successful interventions often require the involvement of multiple parties within the organization. People are much more likely to implement a change if they have a say in its development. An intervention is only a true innovation when change actually takes place in the thinking and behavior of those involved in the professional practice and the practice improves (see also chapter 8 on support).

7.2. Types of Interventions

Interventions can be categorized by the magnitude of the intended changes that can range from small practical changes to modifying existing interventions or practices to designing completely novel approaches.

Minor Interventions

Minor interventions are minimal—but purposeful—changes to everyday practices that are intended to solve a practice problem. For example, adding a question to an intake form, adding to the service schedule by one hour a week, buying more computer terminals for client access, or rearranging the waiting room.

Modifications to Existing Interventions

Significant modifications to existing interventions are required when the design principles suggest the need for substantive changes. You must plan such modifications thoroughly and allocate sufficient time to the design process. You may need to fine-tune the modified interventions by pilot testing and making final adaptations.

> *Example.* A senior center wants to reduce isolation and loneliness among older residents. The staff confer with experienced colleagues at a similar organization about past projects and products that they developed to address this problem. The successful work of the other organization inspires the staff of the senior center to completely redesign their outreach activities to include more home visits and to advertise their services more prominently in the community.

Novel Interventions

When minor interventions do not work and larger changes to existing interventions are also not sufficient, you will have to design a new intervention.

> *Example.* The problem analysis of an agency for youth with drug addictions shows that the relapse rate is higher compared to other agencies. A literature review reveals that peer involvement is a key to relapse prevention. The social workers decide to design a peer involvement program comprised of peer-led support groups and a buddy system. They base the program on the literature review, interviews with staff from other agencies, and interviews with youth receiving services from their agency.

7.3. Design Research Phase 1: Exploratory Research into Design Principles

Design research has two phases. Phase 1 consists of exploratory research in which you complete the key components of orientation, focusing, planning, data collection, and analysis and conclusion to determine the design principles (figure 7.2). The design principles are the qualities that the intervention must possess to solve the practice problem.

The key components of the first design research phase—which are part of the Practitioner Research Cycle and the larger Practitioner Research Method—were discussed at length in the previous chapters. Here we explore them in the context of design research.

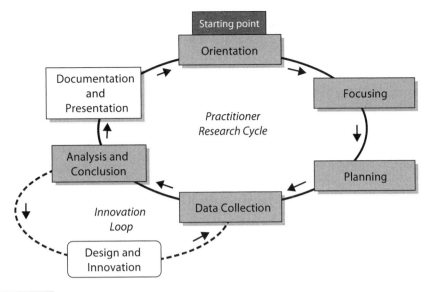

Figure 7.2

Design research phase 1: Exploratory research

Orientation

The orientation phase marks the start of the research process and explores the practice problem. As explained in chapter 3, "practice problem" is a broad term that can encompass gaps or shortcomings within the organization, as well as expectations, opportunities, and challenges for organizations or professionals to keep abreast of new developments. In design research, practice problems can refer to gaps between actual situations and desired situations (Andriessen, 2011; Nieveen & Folmer, 2013) as experienced by various stakeholders. Exploratory problem analysis is therefore always the first step to take.

Focusing

During the focusing stage, you perform an in-depth problem analysis based on a literature review. You then concretize this problem analysis in the formulation of a research objective and research question.

The research question in design research will likely be a derivative of the following question (based on Plomp, 2013):

How can actor (A) in context (B) with target group (C) and with the help of solution (D) achieve output (E)?

Based on the main question, you extrapolate several sub-questions for both research phase 1 (in search of design principles) as well as phase 2 (to create and test the intervention).

Sub-Questions for Research Phase 1

Based on the sub-questions formulated in research phase 1, you shape the design principles required for a successful intervention. You focus on mapping the practice problem as well as on cataloguing the design principles that form the basis for possible solutions (Nieveen & Folmer, 2013). The sub-questions in the first phase of a design study serve different purposes:

Getting to the bottom of the practice problem. During the problem analysis, you gained insight into the practice problem. Sometimes it may be necessary to further deepen your understanding of the practice problem by formulating sub-questions. Answers to such questions can provide insight into possible solutions and be a source for design principles.

Gaining insight into what contributes to the solution of the practice problem according to current theories, opinions of experts, and your professional experience. A design is not only based on the data you collect from your own professional practice, but also on the knowledge found in the practice literature. Therefore, your sub-questions can be aimed at gaining insight from a broader professional perspective. In that way you link your design research to what is already known about the main issues related to your practice problem (Van den Berg & Kouwenhoven, 2008).

Gaining insight into what key stakeholders need and expect related to the solution of the practice problem. You can formulate sub-questions to obtain information required for mapping and clarifying stakeholders' needs, perceptions, and expectations, paying particularly attention to the change they would like to see happen compared to how things are at present (Van den Berg & Kouwenhoven, 2008).

Gaining insight into contextual factors to be considered when designing the solution. You formulate sub-questions that focus on the feasibility of the potential innovation. This leads to design principles focusing on contextual factors that need to be addressed in order to make the intervention successful. These include such factors as time and money but also the support of management and the unwritten rules (organizational culture) regarding how change happens in the organization (Van den Berg & Kouwenhoven, 2008). Some of these factors can be derived from the context analysis.

Sub-Questions for Design Research Phase 2

The sub-questions that you formulate in phase 2 relate to solving the practice problem. The questions focus on intervention design, testing, and evaluating the intervention in the professional practice setting, followed by modifications, if necessary. Sub-questions for research phase 2 will likely be derivatives of the following questions:

What is the most appropriate intervention or design to solve problem X?

After testing, how appropriate (effective) is the intervention or design for solving problem X?

Example. Your practice is interested in enhancing treatment compliance among teenagers diagnosed with insulin-dependent diabetes. Your main research question is how can diabetes nurses enhance treatment compliance of insulin-dependent teenagers from neighborhood X?

Sub-questions for research phase 1:

- In what situations do insulin-dependent teenagers experience low levels of treatment compliance?
- What factors influence treatment compliance of insulin-dependent teenagers?
- How can the contributing factors be modified in order to enhance the treatment compliance of insulin-dependent teenagers?
- What success factors of the project on treatment compliance of elderly people in institution X could possibly also apply to influencing the treatment compliance of insulin-dependent teenagers?
- Which factors need to be considered when striving for greater treatment compliance of insulin-dependent teenagers in neighborhood X?

Sub-questions research phase 2:

- What is the most appropriate intervention or design to enhance therapy compliance of insulin-dependent teenagers from neighborhood X?
- How appropriate or effective is the design after testing?

Planning

During the planning stage, you plot a strategy to execute your design research. Based on your sub-questions for research phase 1, you plan research activities to collect and analyze data that can serve as the basis for formulating design principles (research phase 1). You consider possibilities for testing the intervention in the context of the organization's professional practice (research phase 2). It is advisable to put together a list of colleagues or patients who are willing to help you test the intervention and provide feedback.

Data Collection

You establish the requirements for an effective intervention by collecting data through, for instance, interviews with colleagues, review of specialist literature, observation of patients, and site visits to other organizations that have a successful approach to a similar problem. Your literature review is a main source for creating instruments that help you to systematically and uniformly gather data.

Analysis and Conclusion

Formulating Design Principles

Design principles are the criteria you use for developing an intervention. They are the result of the analysis and conclusion stage, which you have conducted on the data you collected.

> *Example.* A group of therapists researches the interior design and layout requirements for a group therapy room. The following set of design principles was formulated after a patient survey, a review of the literature, a visit to another group therapy space, and interviews with individual therapists.
>
> - Sufficient seating must be available to accommodate the whole group simultaneously.
> - The room must be colorful.
> - The room must be soundproof. Exterior noises must be suppressed inside the room and vice versa.
> - Allergies need to be taken into account in the choice of furnishings.
> - There should be a clear line of sight to other patients from anywhere in the room.
> - There should be an area for quiet contemplation.
> - The maximum budget for the interior design project is $15,000.
>
> These requirements are the design principles that will guide the layout and interior decoration of the group therapy room.

If the principles identified appear not to be feasible, you may be able to gather more information or search for alternatives.

> *Example.* The therapists realize that there is a possible conflict between the requirement of being soundproof and the architecture of the building. They decide to discuss this in more detail with management to explore other solutions to protect the confidentiality of the clients (for example, by using white noise machines).

Once you have obtained a clear overview and definition of the practice problem based on relevant findings from the literature and your own empirical data, you can create a final set of design principles.

Categorizing the Design Principles

Categories help you avoid making errors in defining the practice problem and/or its possible solution. You can base these categories on the categorization you used for formulating sub-questions:

Prior experience and research: literature, experts, other organizations, and personal experience

Stakeholders: the needs and expectations of key stakeholders

Contextual factors: taking into account the specific professional setting

The following category structure for design principles can be applied in numerous situations, as well:

Target group characteristics: size, personal characteristics, abilities or limitations, sociodemographic factors, etc.

Organizational characteristics: available budget, location, employee capacity, and time slots for using the intervention, etc.

Content characteristics: methodology, values, mission of the organization, professional standards, etc.

Example. A maternal and child health center wants to offer the clients a variety of educational opportunities and materials to improve the health and well-being of pregnant women and their children. The center launches a design research project to inform the process. The data is collected through interviews with providers and clients, a site visit to another center, and a review of literature on educational and training programs. The collected data fall under a number of set categories: target group characteristics (level, learning objectives, past endeavors, health care needs), organizational characteristics (duration and frequency of contacts, costs, number of providers), content characteristics (objectives, format, media), and providers' characteristics (level of experience, professional background). The categories help to organize and understand the design principles.

Refining the Design Principles

Clear and unambiguous design principles provide you with a foundation on which to develop the intervention. Vague or imprecise principles are an important reason why interventions fail (Van Aken, 2011). Consider, for instance, the difference between the statements "treatment should not last too long" and "the maximum treatment duration is 20 minutes." The design principles constitute an intervention's most important assessment criteria. Clear phrasing is therefore not only important for intervention design, but also for intervention evaluation.

Example. The following design principles are provided for designing a website to be created by a care facility serving people who are visually impaired:

- All content must be accessible through audio technology.
- The language used must be suitable for both teenage and adult audiences.
- The site needs to offer content for specific target groups: adults, youth, service providers, and family/friends.

Substantiating the Design Principles

It is important to explain what data have led to the formulation of each individual design principle.

Example. A support program for homeless youth keeps a record of textual sources, interviews with the youth, and site visits as a way to substantiate design principles surrounding the following research question: "How should program staff approach homeless youth to make them aware of their personal strengths and abilities?"

Design principles	Which data forms the basis for this design principle?
Dialogue techniques used by counselors should make homeless youth become aware of their personal strengths and abilities.	*Textual source*: Anish et al. (2014) confirmed the efficacy of the Social Competence Model for enhancing the social competence of adolescents. *Interview with a homeless youth*: Joe indicates that in the past he was frequently confronted with failure. By talking with program staff, he was able to recognize his strengths and abilities. *Textual source*: The mission statement drafted by the board on March 12, 2014, explicitly names a strengths-based approach as being the basis for all assistance provided.
The issues that homeless youth are facing should be identified and addressed as early as possible.	*Textual sources*: "According to providers, assessing immediate needs is a primary focus when young people enter crisis programs" (National Alliance to End Homelessness, 2015, p. 7). "Providers also stressed the importance of developing capacity within schools to intervene quickly with minor youth in crisis. Stabilizing services at that point could prevent both homelessness and a disrupted education." (National Alliance to End Homelessness, 2015, p. 3). Homeless youth indicate many improvements are needed in social services. One remarkable fact is that 80 percent of homeless youth are very satisfied with their personal counselors. On the other hand, 85 percent also indicate that help at an earlier stage is preferable and, in their case, would have likely had a positive impact (Reed Business, 2010). *Group interview with social workers*: "We notice that many young people do not know how to deal with their problems. They are in desperate need of help in this respect."
Homeless youth should only have to deal with a limited number of professionals.	*Textual sources*: "Providers said they are concerned that, if not addressed, the issues that led youth to seek shelter may resurface when they return home. Therefore they seek to create sustainable family connections to ongoing financial, behavioral health care, and other supports" (National Alliance to End Homelessness, 2015, p. 7). The feedback we hear is that social assistance lacks continuity. Fifty percent [of homeless youth] have lived in two to five care facilities (Reed Business, 2010). That is a very unsettling life. *Site visit to comparable facility*: The site visit showed that the majority of youth had a maximum of two regular counselors. This was named as being very important by 12 out of 13 youths.

Sources: K. R. Anish, G. S. Divya, & S. M. Skaria, 2014, Social competence model for adolescents: Reflections from an intervention study, *Artha Journal of Social Sciences, 13*(2), 1–19; National Alliance to End Homelessness, 2015, *Ending homelessness for unaccompanied minor youth*, https://endhomelessness.org /resource/ending-homelessness-for-unaccompanied-minor-youth; Reed Business, 2010, Timely help to homeless youth makes the difference [in Dutch], *Zorg+Welzijn*, https://www.zorgwelzijn.nl/vroege-hulp -aan-zwerfjongeren-maakt-het-verschil-zwz015597w.

Feedback from Stakeholders

Asking the stakeholders (e.g., colleagues, patients/clients) to review the list of design principles prior to creating the intervention is advisable for the following reasons:

- Your analysis of the practice problem is validated by those who will implement and use the intervention.
- Direct involvement of the stakeholders in the creative process increases internal support for your intervention.
- You build a sense of ownership. Implementation is facilitated when stakeholders can identify with the intervention; it is more likely that the organization will adopt your intervention and subsequently promote internal change through its use.
- Your design process becomes transparent. Stakeholders can clearly see what steps you took to reach the final intervention.

Exercise 1. Formulating Design Principles (see page 227)

7.4. Research Phase 2: Innovation Loop

The Innovation Loop of phase 2 is where you develop the intervention based on the design principles you formulated in phase 1 (figure 7.3). You then test your intervention in the professional setting by collecting and analyzing data during the implementation. Based on the conclusions, you can decide on possibly modifying and retesting the intervention. Hence, you complete the Innovation Loop (which exists only in design research) once or multiple times. Once the intervention proves effective in practice, you document the research and present your final intervention design.

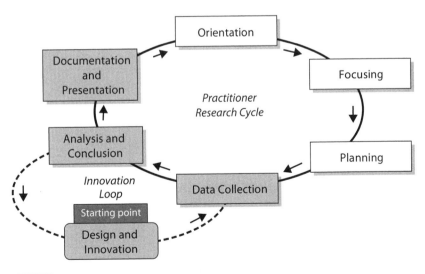

Figure 7.3

Design research phase 2: Innovation Loop

Designing is both a systematic and creative process. In the following sections, we discuss the key components within the Innovation Loop, which you can launch after you have formulated clear design principles for the intervention.

Key Component: Design and Innovation

If you know what design principles your innovation requires, you can think about designing an intervention that can provide a solution to your practice problem. It is important that you first generate multiple design ideas and then choose the one that is most suitable. Even when you have very clear design principles, there might be countless ideas about potential innovations that could solve the problem. Let yourself explore several different possibilities before settling on one alternative by following these three steps: generate multiple design ideas, make a reasoned decision for the most appropriate solution, and create one prototype design to test.

Step 1: Generate Design Ideas

To generate design ideas, you need to use creative techniques that stimulate *divergent thinking*, which means opening ourselves to exploring many possible solutions. Think, for example, of techniques that are presented in other chapters of this book, such as brainstorming, mind mapping, concept mapping, perspective change, and freewriting. Instead of generating or exploring practice problems or questions, you are now using these techniques to generate design ideas. Based on the design principles and your own creative power, you generate various design ideas that can contribute to solving the problem.

Design ideas can be based on different forms of interventions. Several common forms are discussed in this section. This list is not exhaustive, but rather serves as a source of inspiration.

Informational material

Professionals often make extensive use of informational material on topics such as substance abuse, depression, safety at home, autism, or services available to mothers and children. When designing these resources, consider such aspects as the objectives in providing the material, content, context (where and how distributed), language, and medium.

Assignments

Assignments, or tasks, are used to help (groups of) patients or clients learn new skills or gain knowledge, express thoughts and emotions, or engage in community activities. These tasks or exercises can be offered on paper, digitally, orally, or online. Examples of possible assignments are collaborative projects to enhance group cohesion, exercises to enhance client/patient self-reliance, or role-plays to prepare clients for a job interview. You need to define the learning objectives in detail and have a clear view of the social, cognitive, and emotional context of the clients/patients before you embark on the intervention design process.

Expert systems

Expert systems aim to make knowledge widely available within the organization or between organizations. An example of the latter is a knowledge base on health care and social support for local district nurses and other primary care workers. Your design process would focus on presentation, content, and interaction potential, for example.

Job aids

Job aids have a twofold function: on the one hand, they promote knowledge dispersion within the organization; on the other hand, they act as a framework for professional conduct. Examples include guidelines for training new employees, brochures on counseling patients who have lost a loved one, or instruction manuals for medical equipment.

Interior design and layout

The layout of common rooms, workspaces, or waiting areas undoubtedly plays a role in health care and social work settings. A conversation while seated on opposite sides of a table will likely be different from talking to one another on a sofa. Factors you include in the layout and design of spaces are, for instance, furniture arrangements, color, natural light, materials, room to maneuver, and privacy. You can design changes to the layout of existing rooms or the interior design of new spaces on paper, using 3D software, or in scale models first. The latter gives the people involved a concrete impression of what the design will look like in reality. This way, colleagues, patients/clients, and board members can evaluate your intervention design and give you feedback.

Public relations materials

You can keep patients, clients, parents, colleagues, or other parties informed through brochures, leaflets, newsletters, and websites. Each PR product has a clear communication objective, such as stimulating clients to sign up for courses, fundraising, encouraging parents or guardians to join a committee, or informing other service providers about new services.

Instruments for testing and evaluation

The health care and social work sectors make extensive use of test and evaluation instruments. Many of the instruments used are standardized tests that were developed after extensive research over long periods of time to evaluate a client/patient's problem or to assess the effectiveness of services. Existing instruments often need to be adapted to other specific practice settings. Where there is no instrument available that meets your needs, you will need to develop your own.

Practice methods and techniques

You and your health care and social work colleagues employ different methods and techniques in your work. Professional practice is guided by the ethics and norms of one's profession. But a professional decision always needs to take into account the specifics of the situation at hand, considering both the abilities and wishes of the patient/client as well as one's own experience as a practitioner. In design research, you can focus on developing new or modifying existing practice methods and techniques tailored to your specific practice setting.

Systems for planning, administration, and registration

A regular workday sees a lot of administrative work, such as logs of completed tasks, chart notes, updates to patient files, daily planning, and minutes of meetings. Many of these administrative tasks follow an internal protocol or format and often make use of electronic systems that can be adapted to different user requirements or profiles. In design research, you can focus, for instance, on redesigning your electronic health record system to better meet the needs of staff and regulatory requirements.

Exercise 2. Generating and Selecting Design Ideas (see page 228)

Step 2: Make a Reasoned Decision for the Most Appropriate Solution

When selecting design ideas, you take a *convergent* approach. You critically assess the various design ideas that you have generated for the purpose of reducing them to what you would like to focus on. Your design principles will serve as the main criteria for this process. Additionally, Plomp et al. (1992) provide the following list of general requirements for selecting the intervention (the best solution) for a practice problem. The intervention should be

- sufficiently detailed,
- user-friendly,
- acceptable to all users, and
- realistic in terms of the time and resources required.

You can apply one of the following four techniques to select the most appropriate solution:

Technique 1: Weighted decision matrix

You can reach a decision on the final intervention design by *weighing* the pros and cons of the different options (Vos, 1992). You can perform this activity alone or in cooperation with other stakeholders.

Example. Your research question is "How can the coordinators in a rehabilitation center tailor daily activities to patients' interests?" The following design principles came from your exploratory research (research phase 1):

1. Preparation of the activities should not take more than 15 minutes per patient per week.
2. The intervention should provide a solution allowing the patients to engage in different activities each week.
3. The activities should be in line with the patients' interests.
4. The range of activities should stimulate patients to make their own choices.

Given these principles, you have chosen to compare two design ideas based on three criteria:

Intervention idea	Does the intervention fit the design principles?	Does the intervention solve the practice problem?	Is the intervention feasible and realistic?
A rotation system with different activities each day. Patients can pick daily activities from a weekly changing selection.	The intervention fits the principles, but the question remains if the activity coordinators will have time to come up with a new range of activities every week. Patients may also choose the same activity repeatedly.	The intervention seems to be a good solution to the practice problem.	The intervention requires a very extensive range of activities and materials. Quite a lot of preparation is involved, as well as a significant investment in materials.
Give each week a different theme, with corresponding activities from which the patients may choose.	The intervention complies with design principles 1 and 2, but patients may not always be offered activities that suit their interests.	As the interests of the patients are not at the center of this intervention, it does not seem to be a solution to the practice problem.	The intervention does not pose any organizational issues.

Using this matrix, you can quickly see the pros and cons of the two intervention ideas. The first idea provides a solution to the practice problem, but it requires more preparation and logistical arrangements. The second idea is easier to implement while it provides only a partial solution to the problem. In practitioner research, you often need to make decisions based on your resources and the context.

Technique 2: Reverse brainstorming

This technique focuses on generating points of criticism rather than ideas (Vos, 1992). A group of stakeholders looks at the list of design ideas and formulates points of criticism based on the design principles. The group then tries to revise the design ideas by addressing the problems identified. The design idea that, after revision, meets the design principles best and also seems to solve the problem will probably be the most appropriate solution.

Technique 3: Idea advocate

In contrast to the previous technique, an "idea advocate" presents all the design ideas to a group of interested stakeholders, highlighting the advantages of each design by taking into account the design principles (Vos, 1992). After all design ideas have been presented, the group chooses the one they feel is the best solution.

Technique 4: Nominal technique

The nominal technique, described in chapter 5, can also be used when choosing a design idea. Each participant chooses the design ideas that they think are most appropriate, taking into account the design principles. Each group member presents his or her choices to the group. The choices of all group members are displayed together in the form of a list. Each group member then choose three topics from this list and rates them with one, two, or three points. The design idea with the most points will likely be the most appropriate solution.

Step 3: Create the Design

After conferring with the stakeholders and making a well-founded choice, you can work out the details of the intervention design. The preliminary version of your design is called a *prototype* (Van den Berg & Kouwenhoven, 2008).

Key Component: Data Collection

After you have created the prototype, you test it in practice by conducting a pilot study. You can use one or several testing strategies, but depending on the nature of the intervention, patients/clients and/or staff members may need some form of preparation in advance. When you test a prototype, you are conducting a *formative* or *intermediate* evaluation for the purpose of creating an improved, final version of the intervention that can be implemented in practice (Van den Akker & Thijs, 2009).

You have two objectives when testing the intervention. The first is assessing compliance with the design principles, which determines to what extent the stakeholders feel that the intervention complies in practice with the previously formulated design principles.

> *Example.* A maternity ward faces high patient dissatisfaction. Research into the issue shows, in part, that patients are very dissatisfied with the lack of privacy. Young mothers feel that they are always in plain view, that the ward is overpopulated, and that noise levels are too high. A set of design principles is created in cooperation with the stakeholders (patients and staff) to address this problem. A prototype for an intervention is developed that addresses the layout of the ward, visiting hours, seating arrangements, and noise levels. Patients and nursing staff evaluate these changes based on assessment questions that are derived from the design principles.

Your second objective is to formulate new or additional design principles should (part of) the first set of design principles prove to be inadequate, incorrectly formulated, or irrelevant. It is important to gather data not only on the design principles but also on user experience. Where were the difficulties? Are there suggestions for modifications? Do the users have any other relevant input?

Testing Strategies

Several strategies are at your disposal for testing the intervention in practice (Nieveen & Folmer, 2013). The professional context as well as the size and scope of the intervention determine which testing strategy is most suitable. If the Innovation Loop will be conducted repeatedly (several rounds of testing and improving your design), it is advisable to apply the test strategies in phases.

Rating checklist

This strategy uses a printed checklist to collect data. Those involved rate the degree to which the intervention fulfills each of the design principles.

Focus group

This strategy relies on interviews to collect data. You present a small group of those involved in the intervention to discuss the pros and cons based on statements or questions that you provide. Variety in the participants' perspectives (patients/clients, staff, management) ensures a multifaceted evaluation of the intervention.

Walk-through

This strategy relies on questions and observations to collect data. You go over the steps of the intervention with those involved to elicit feedback on each component and how it was implemented for the purpose if collecting detailed data on how the intervention functioned.

Small-scale testing

Here you test the intervention with a limited group of colleagues or patients/clients to collect data. The intervention is only implemented on a large scale in the organization when all the design principles are met.

Example. A social service center experiments with vouchers that unemployed clients can use to try out several lines of work for a short period of time under the supervision of a job coach. This structure enables the employer and (potential) employee to get to know each other without the need for a commitment. Initially, the pilot involves only a limited number of companies and unemployed individuals. After the pilot test, a decision will be taken on whether the vouchers will be introduced on a larger scale.

Testing parts of the intervention

Sometimes it is useful to test parts of your intervention separately. For example, when designing a new service consisting of an intake procedure, a treatment, and a follow-up, you could test each of these components separately to assess how each component reflects the design principles and contributes to solving the problem. Once all components have been evaluated and modified, they can be brought together for a full implementation of the intervention.

Full implementation

Full implementation means that the entire intervention is put into practice for the whole organization. The advantage of this approach is that the intervention as intended is tested. The disadvantage is that large-scale change is implemented in the organization without knowing if it will be successful.

Exercise 3. **Testing and Data Collection** (see page 228)

Key Component: Analysis and Conclusion

In pilot-testing your intervention, you are analyzing the data you collected according to the following criteria:

1. Does the intervention comply with the design principles?
2. Has testing the intervention uncovered new issues that need to be addressed in the intervention design?

If the answer to the first question is yes, and the answer to the second question is no, your intervention will largely perform adequately in practice and, for the most part, solve the practice problem. If your intervention does indeed solve the practice problem, you can conclude the research project by completing the last key component, documentation and presentation, which includes reporting on the final version of your intervention.

If the answer to the first question is no or the answer to the second question is yes, however, you will have to repeat the Innovation Loop.

The Intervention Does Not Comply with the Design Principles

If the analysis leads to the conclusion that those involved feel that the intervention insufficiently meets the design principles, you need to modify the intervention design. Make sure the negative feedback is not merely a symptom of resistance to change. View feedback as a positive expression of involvement. People need to get used to this new way of doing things, so allocate sufficient time for testing and provide for a supportive environment during the testing phase.

New Design Principles Arise

Testing your intervention may lead to new insights regarding the practice problem or uncover new issues. If this is the case, you must adjust the design principles, and it is important that you highlight the new insights that led to a new interpretation of the practice problem.

> *Example.* The students who receive after-school tutoring at a social service agency have problems concentrating because the tutoring space is also used for recreational purposes. The agency's research into the issue leads to a new layout for the office space, with privacy rooms for studying. Evaluation of the new layout at a later stage reveals another issue: It is not just the space that influences the students' concentration, but also problems in how the students are being tutored. The students need an intensified one-on-one support. Training for tutors is added to the intervention design.

The process of modifying the intervention is also called *redesign*. You essentially complete the Innovation Loop again, while at the same time collecting new data. You answer the two analysis questions using that data and repeat this process until your intervention complies with the design principles and no new issues arise.

However, redesigning an intervention cannot go on forever. It is simply not always possible to align the design principles 100 percent with the needs of the organization. Concessions will sometimes have to be made—especially for time-sensitive interventions.

Key Component: Documentation and Presentation

Once you have finalized your intervention, you conclude the design research with a report and a presentation of your most important findings. Part of this process began earlier in the research, when colleagues helped you with the creation and testing of your intervention. This process provided them with partial insight into your activities and the results of your research. The research report documents and explains both the steps and the decisions that you took in the research process. In the report, you detail the path that led to the first intervention design (prototype) and to any subsequent modifications.

Embedding the results of your research in the organization's practices is an important part of this final key component. Consider the following aspects:

Intervention Assimilation

The design research was your first step in persuading the organization to adopt your intervention. True innovation success is achieved by complete integration of your intervention into the organization's practices. Even after completing the design research, you need to schedule further implementation steps and put forward other suggestions for adoption of the intervention if it is to become an integral part of the organization (see chapter 8).

Long-Term Effects of the Intervention (Summative Evaluation)

Formative evaluation during the design process provided you with insight into the practical application of the intervention. You made modifications to the intervention design based on the data that you collected. But the effectiveness of the intervention cannot always be determined in the time it takes to complete the research cycle. Some effects may only become visible in the long term, once the intervention has been integrated into practice for some time. Determining the effectiveness of an intervention is achieved by way of a *summative* or *final evaluation* (Nieveen & Folmer, 2013). Summative evaluations can become part of the regular quality assurance cycles of the organization (depending on the scope and level of the intervention). Such an evaluation can firmly embed the results of your design research within the organization.

> *Example.* A supervised program for teenagers diagnosed with Type I diabetes that was developed by nurses in the diabetes department of a hospital three years ago includes peer-to-peer sessions as one of its integral components. In the context of a summative evaluation, the group of nurses is now researching the effects of the program on treatment compliance. To determine if the program needs adjustments, the findings are compared to research that was carried out four years prior.

Exercise 4. Implementation Strategies (see page 228)

7.5. Rapid Prototyping

There is a design methodology with a heavy emphasis on testing and evaluation known as *rapid prototyping* (Tripp & Bichelmeyer, 1990). The term "evolutionary prototyping" is also used for this method, the origins of which lie in the technology sector. In rapid prototyping, the first phase of the design research process is composed of the activities, which are conducted in a short period of time. Early in the second research phase a first draft (prototype) of the intervention is created. Data on the possibilities and limitations of the intervention are acquired quickly by testing and evaluating the prototype with the stakeholders. The prototype is modified, and another evaluation round follows. The Innovation Loop is completed several times. To minimize the effects of trial and error, it is important to link the prototype to the practice problem, testing and evaluating it frequently and systematically. Equally important is the process of documenting the design principles and substantiating them based on theory and practice.

This methodology is preferable if

- tangible results are required in a short period of time,
- the method suits the organizational culture,
- decisions on the required resources/investments must be taken soon,
- stakeholders cannot grasp the practice problem fully or imagine a solution,
- not much information on the practice problem is provided in the literature, or
- it is to be expected that the problem and the solution may be identified more quickly through prototyping.

Example. Team leaders are interested in the use of "care bots" to help alleviate the feelings of loneliness in elderly patients. Both patients and patient counselors have difficulty defining how these robots can provide added value, as they find it difficult to picture the robots in use. The team leaders decide to test the care bots in practice and systematically collect assessment data. This information forms the basis for their design principles.

7.6. Summary

This chapter discussed the steps you take in design research in order to create a successful intervention design, as well as how you test the intervention in professional practice. Three degrees of intervention are distinguished: minor interventions regarding the practice's daily routine or environment, modifying an existing intervention, and designing a completely novel intervention (innovation).

Design research is essentially split into two research phases. During the exploratory first phase, you complete the key components of orientation, focusing, planning, data collection, and analysis and conclusion in order to determine the design principles for an effective intervention to solve the practice problem (prototype). In the second research phase, you complete the Innovation Loop once or several times. Only in design research is the Innovation Loop part of the Practitioner Research Method.

The Innovation Loop starts off with the key component of design and innovation, which consists of the following steps:

- Finding resources and choosing an intervention form
- Developing the intervention
- Planning intervention tests

You employ one or several strategies to test the intervention. During the test period, you collect data in order to perform a formative evaluation of your intervention. You check compliance of the intervention with the existing design principles and identify missing design principles. Those involved in the intervention (clients/patients, staff, management) are an important source of information. If your intervention does not meet the design principles or if new design principles are identified, you complete the Innovation Loop once more. You redesign and test your intervention, conducting a formative evaluation. You repeat this process until your intervention complies with the design principles and no new issues arise. In the next steps, you document your findings in a research report, present the final intervention, and implement the intervention in the professional context. Once your intervention is implemented, you can perform a summative evaluation at a later stage to observe the long-term effects.

Rapid prototyping is a design methodology with a heavy emphasis on repeated testing and evaluation within a short period of time.

EXERCISES

Exercise 1. Formulating Design Principles

Formulate a set of possible design principles that could guide the development of the following interventions:

- A device to help people with a visual impairment to cook
- A protocol for lifting and carrying patients
- A redesign of the organization's website
- The layout of the consultation zone of the staff area
- Procedures for training new staff
- An intake interview procedure
- The curriculum of a school-based sexual abuse prevention program
- A project aimed at teaching youth to manage their money
- Portrait painting as a therapeutic activity for patients with a mental health issues

Exercise 2. Generating and Selecting Design Ideas

Generate as many different design ideas as possible for the example here (or an example from your own practice). Use one or more techniques from this book. Then use the weighted decision technique to determine which design idea best meets the design principles.

> *Example.* A social welfare organization in the inner city wants to alleviate loneliness among older residents. Their design principles include:
> - Each person must experience at least one social interaction on a daily basis.
> - The social welfare organization can monitor the clients' reaction to the interaction.
> - Both mobile and less mobile persons are to be served.

Exercise 3. Testing and Data Collection

Several testing strategies were presented in this chapter. Give an example of how each strategy can be applied to the following intervention (or an intervention of your choosing): A new digital patient registration system structured in such a way that staff notes can be added and patient files can be accessed remotely.

Exercise 4. Implementation Strategies

Consider the innovations that have recently been implemented in your organization or in an organization that you are familiar with. Which implementation strategies were used? Which other implementation strategies could have been used as well or instead?

REFERENCES

Andriessen, D. (2011). Veldprobleem, kennisprobleem, deelvragen [Field problem, knowledge problem, sub-questions]. In J. van Aken & D. Andriessen (Eds.), *Handboek ontwerpgericht wetenschappelijk onderzoek: Wetenschap met effect* [Handbook on design-focused scientific research: Science with effect] (pp. 119–127). Boom Lemma.

Nieveen, N., & Folmer, E. (2013). Formative evaluation in educational design research. In T. Plomp & N. Nieveen (Eds.), *Educational design research part A: An introduction* (pp. 152–169). SLO.

Plomp, T. (2013). Educational design research: An introduction. In T. Plomp & N. Nieveen (Eds.), *Educational design research part A: An introduction* (pp. 10–51). SLO.

Plomp, T., Feteris, A., Pieters, J. M., & Tomic, W. (1992). *Ontwerpen van onderwijs en trainingen* [Designing educational programs and training courses]. Lemma.

Tripp, S., & Bichelmeyer, B. (1990). Rapid prototyping: An alternative instructional design strategy. *Educational Technology Research and Development, 38*(1), 31–44. https://doi.org/10.1007/BF02298246

Van Aken, J. (2011). Domeinonafhankelijke ontwerptheorie [Domain-independent design theory]. In J. van Aken & D. Andriessen (Eds.), *Handboek ontwerpgericht wetenschappelijk onderzoek: Wetenschap met effect* [Handbook on design-focused scientific research: Science with effect] (pp. 41–59). Boom Lemma.

Van den Akker, J., & Thijs, A. (2009). *Leerplan in ontwikkeling* [Curriculum in development]. SLO.

Van den Berg, E., & Kouwenhoven, W. (2008). Ontwerponderzoek in vogelvlucht [Design research in a nutshell]. *Tijdschrift voor Lerarenopleiders* [Journal for Teacher Educators], *29*(4), 20–26.

Van Leeuwen, S. (2004). Innoveren in de thuiszorg vraagt om een kritische aanpak [Innovating in home care requires a critical approach]. *Zorgspecial* [Health Care Special] *6*(4), 1–4.

Vos, H. J. (1992). Het kiezen van een oplossing [Choosing a solution]. In T. Plomp et al. (Eds.), *Ontwerpen van onderwijs en trainingen* [Designing educational programs and training courses] (pp. 195–220). Lemma.

Documentation and Presentation

I n practitioner research, various stakeholders are involved during all stages of the research project. You should be thinking about documentation and presentation throughout your research project as an important part of reflecting on your work and creating support for the research activities and the results (figure 8.1). In this last phase of practitioner research, you will share your findings not only with the stakeholders who were involved in your work but also with third parties who may have an interest in the study.

Chapter 8 introduces effective tools and methods of dissemination and implementation of research results. The characteristics and interests of the target audience play a major role in planning research activities. In addition, selecting an appropriate communication strategy to disseminate the findings in the form of a report and/or other types of presentation is important, as well as highlighting implementation strategies for affecting positive changes using the research data. Topics such as evaluation of the research, reflection, and future recommendations are explored here. The chapter concludes with a brief summary and relevant exercises.

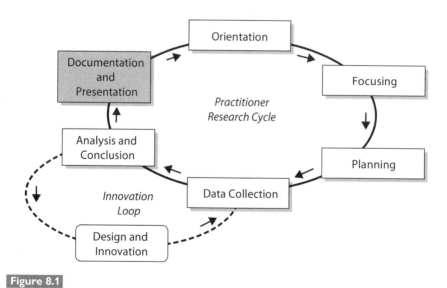

Figure 8.1

Key components of practitioner research: Documentation and Presentation

8.1. Dissemination and Implementation of the Findings

"The research is almost done; all that is left is presenting the findings to my colleagues." This statement oversimplifies the challenge of dissemination and implementation. You must first identify the audience for your findings, which may extend well beyond your immediate colleagues. Then you carefully assess their needs and other characteristics (i.e., their sociodemographic and disciplinary backgrounds). The next step is to consider, based on the objectives of your research, whether your primary focus is on spreading the knowledge gained in the study (dissemination) or on putting the findings into practice (implementation).

Dissemination is relevant when generating new knowledge and insights is the central research objective (section 8.3). Your communication strategy will consist of enhancing awareness and spreading new knowledge among your audience.

> *Example.* A dental hygienist is interested in researching the needs of anxious patients. Her study identifies both characteristics of patients as well as ways of practicing that contribute to the anxiety. She writes up her central findings and distributes them to everyone in her practice and also presents them at a conference on dental medicine.

Implementation is relevant when the research objective is developing a new way of doing practice (applying innovations). Davis and Taylor-Vaisey (1997) state that this requires effective communication strategies as well as educational and policy-related techniques to remove obstacles to change. As the researcher who developed and tested the innovation, you can provide support during the implementation process, even if you are not directly responsible for instituting the change.

> *Example.* In the context of her research, a dental hygienist creates and tests a protocol for how to treat anxious patients. Additionally, she asks a number of her colleagues to test the protocol and provide feedback. The protocol is established as a new standard for practice in the dental clinic, with the dental hygienist who executed the research at the helm of the implementation process.

8.2. Identifying the Target Audience

You must determine what individuals or groups your target audience comprises prior to making decisions on strategies for communicating your findings and implementing possible changes. The target audience is not always one homogenous group nor necessarily the same as the group of stakeholders who participated in your research (see chapter 4). Thus, you must consider the scope and diversity of the target group.

Example 1. When assessing various forms of communication between local groups of adolescents, various stakeholders are involved. A group of adolescents comprise your research population. Colleagues are consulted in designing and helping you to carry out your research. Your management provides support and also advice on how to proceed. Your target audience can include all of these stakeholders as well as social work professionals and local policy makers interested in the topic under study.

Example 2. In a practitioner research project, several family counselors are interviewed about their preferred methods of working with families. These counselors form both the research population and the target audience. Additionally, the board of the organization where the family counselors work may also be part of the target audience.

You as the Audience

Earlier in the book, we stated that practitioner research may be conducted solely for the benefit of the practitioner researcher. For example, you might research the way in which you promote patient interaction in a discussion group, and the results provide you with principles to enhance patient interaction during group activities in the future. In this case, you as the researcher are the sole member of the target audience. Even if the research is primarily being conducted for your benefit, however, we recommend that you prepare the results in such a way that they are also comprehensible for others. You may want to share your findings at some point in the future.

Various Other Target Audiences

Research often applies to several target audiences at once. For example, a manual is written and tested in practice by a graduate student nurse addressing the cultural diversity of patients. The target audiences for this research include fellow nurses, patients and their relatives, supervisors, nurse educators, and fellow graduate students. Each target audience has a different interest in the research results. For some groups, presenting the research design and findings might be sufficient, while others need to be actively involved in the implementation of new work methods.

While identifying target audiences, you often need to distinguish between three types:

Primary target group(s): persons for whom the research results have a direct impact. These are often clients/patients and colleagues.

Secondary target group(s): persons who are not directly affected by the research results but who need to be informed. Think, for example, of relatives of clients/patients, board members, or colleagues from other locations.

Intermediate target group(s): persons or organizations that play a critical role in communicating the research and translating it into products, policies, and programs, such as management, policy makers, editors of professional journals, professional networks, and the like.

Table 8.1. Social map created by a nursing student to identify various target audiences and their areas of interest relevant to her practitioner research	
Target audience	Relevant areas of interest
Nurses (primary target group)	Gaining new insights and knowledge on how to adapt their nursing home's daily routine and practices to patients' socioeconomic backgrounds.
Management (primary target group)	Learning important details about the research process and results, especially those related to the benefits and consequences of the research regarding changes in practice or policy.
University professors (secondary target group)	Demonstrating the personal and professional development of the nursing student with respect to course requirements.
Editorial board of a professional journal (intermediate target group)	Examining the validity of the results and potential usefulness of the study for publication.

Consider the differences between the various target audiences when documenting and presenting the research, as well as when implementing changes (table 8.1). This is a *social mapping* exercise that needs to be conducted in order to plan relevant dissemination and implementation activities (Grol et al., 2013).

One Target Audience with Subgroups

Even within a homogenous group (such as occupational therapists or a management team), differences may exist between subgroups of members (Grol et al., 2013). Some subgroups may be more reluctant to change their practice, while others may be more interested in promoting new developments.

When analyzing the characteristics of target groups, you can identify subgroups by paying attention to the similarities and differences regarding the following:

- Demographic or personal characteristics such as age, level of education, language, gender, and occupation.
- Problem-related (or domain-specific) characteristics such as their current knowledge about the subject, work experience, and the involvement and expectations regarding the proposed solution.

Each target group and subgroup within a target group may have different interests in the results of the research. When reporting and presenting your research and implementing changes, try to consider such differences as much as possible.

Four basic dissemination strategies can be broadly categorized using a *communication matrix* (Van Ruler, 1998) that considers your communication objective (table 8.2). The objectives range from simply sharing findings to influencing the target audience and from only sending information to sending and receiving information. With these objectives in mind, dissemination strategies boil down to the following options:

Information: a controlled one-way form of communication. In the context of the health care and social work sectors, this occurs when research results are presented in a meeting, at a conference, or in a newsletter. The main objective is to inform the audience.

Dialogue: a two-way form of communication that values the input of the stakeholders. In health care and social work settings, this approach is often found at staff meetings, in supervision, and in case consultations. Practitioner research findings can be shared in the context of a dialogue in order to produce feedback on the meaning of the findings for practice.

Persuasion: a form of one-way communication focused on influencing the opinion or actions of the target audience. The findings of practitioner research can be communicated in such a way as to convince the audience of the need to make changes, showing the shortfalls of current practice and options for the future.

Building consensus: both the researcher and the audience are engaged in communication about the research findings in order to determine together the meaning of the research for practice.

Example. A group of youth workers has conducted a practitioner research project on the question of how local youth can be motivated to enhance the livability of their neighborhood. In the research project, the workers have collaborated closely with a group of local youth. In a final meeting, they present the results of their research and organize a world café session to generate ideas for dissemination of the results in the neighborhood (*dialogue*). The workers discuss these results in a workshop with their colleagues to come to a shared view on the final dissemination and implementation plan (*building consensus*). Next, they present the research results together with the dissemination and implementation plan to the city council for the purpose of obtaining financial support (*persuasion*). Finally, they give a presentation of their findings at a conference for social work (*informing*).

Exercise 1. Communication Matrix (see page 249)

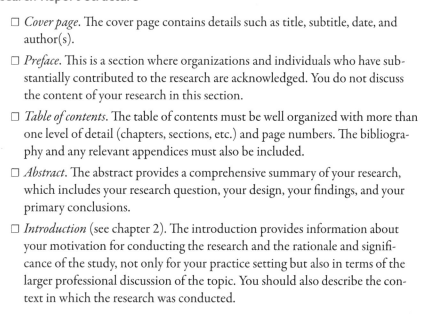

Table 8.2. Using a communication matrix template to identify specific communication strategies based on communication objectives		
	Sharing findings	Influencing the target audience
Sending information only	Information	Persuasion
Sending and receiving information	Dialogue	Building consensus

Documentation

Practitioner research contributes in various degrees to the development of the organization in which it takes place and also to the advancement of professional knowledge. Documentation is a general requirement for internal quality assurance, transparency, and external accountability. It is therefore vital that you deliver a clear and well-founded research report. The research report lends credibility to your research. When you disseminate the report, make a choice to either inform or persuade the audience. A report based on a process of dialogue or building consensus will reflect the views not only of the researcher but of others as well.

Choose the form and scope of documentation and presentation that best suits your research objective and the target audience. This may mean using different forms for different target audiences or subgroups. The report can be comprised solely of text, or you can make use of new technologies, such as interactive online tools or audiovisual elements. Research reports often follow a generic structure similar to the one we describe here. If you are wanting to publish your results on an online platform or in a journal, keep in mind that each has its own formatting and submission requirements that are usually posted on the their websites.

Research Report Structure

- ☐ *Cover page.* The cover page contains details such as title, subtitle, date, and author(s).
- ☐ *Preface.* This is a section where organizations and individuals who have substantially contributed to the research are acknowledged. You do not discuss the content of your research in this section.
- ☐ *Table of contents.* The table of contents must be well organized with more than one level of detail (chapters, sections, etc.) and page numbers. The bibliography and any relevant appendices must also be included.
- ☐ *Abstract.* The abstract provides a comprehensive summary of your research, which includes your research question, your design, your findings, and your primary conclusions.
- ☐ *Introduction* (see chapter 2). The introduction provides information about your motivation for conducting the research and the rationale and significance of the study, not only for your practice setting but also in terms of the larger professional discussion of the topic. You should also describe the context in which the research was conducted.

- *Problem definition* (see chapters 2 and 3). The problem definition contains a description of the practice problem, the results of the literature review, as well as the research objectives and research questions.

- *Method* (see chapters 4 and 5). The methods section contains a description of your methods of data collection and analysis. You should reference the literature sources you used to guide your choice and application of methods. If possible, specify which methods you applied to each of the research questions. This section also includes a description of how you involved stakeholders in your research.

- *Ethical considerations*. Describe the ethical issues raised by your research and how you addressed them, including informed consent, confidentiality, and anonymity.

- *Findings* (see chapters 6 and 7). This section contains the most important results of your data analysis (preferably categorized by sub-question), but you do not attach conclusions to these findings. If you carry out design research, you present a brief description of the intervention. You can include a complete intervention description in the appendices.

- *Conclusion* (see chapter 6). The conclusion contains your answers to the main research question, and to the sub-questions, where applicable. You also state your recommendations for practice based on your findings. In your answer to the research question, you indicate to what extent your research solved the practice problem. Demonstrate a clear connection between the conclusion(s) and the results of the analysis that you presented in the findings section.

- *Discussion* (see section 8.5). In this section, the findings and your conclusions are discussed in the context of the research literature and the larger professional discussion of the problem. You judge the strength and validity of your research by reporting potential limitations, challenges, and other critical points regarding the execution of the research. When appropriate, make suggestions for future research and describe the dissemination and implementation strategy.

- *Bibliography* (see appendix for details)

- *Appendices*. An appendix can contain, for example, the instruments that you used for data collection (such as interview questions and written questionnaires), a detailed description of the final intervention (for design research), raw data (such as detailed reports or transcripts of interview and data tables for quantitative results), self-reflection reports, and an implementation plan. You do not necessarily need to include all of this material in the appendix, however. Your setting and your dissemination strategy will help you determine what to include.

Tips for Composing the Research Report

Considerations in the following categories may help you to write your research report (based on Altrichter et al., 2008; Hall, 2013; World Wide Writing, 2019):

Outlining

- Create a detailed outline for the structure of your research report before you start the writing process. In a few lines or key words, name and describe the function of each component of the report as well as the intended content (table 8.3).

Selecting data

- You decide which part of the substantial amount of collected data you will include in the research report, based on its relevance to the research question.
- Explain how you dealt with any missing data (see chapter 6).

Ethical issues

- If you have made agreements with participants regarding anonymity, you must safeguard their privacy and the secure storage of the data.
- All data that identifies specific persons or organizations requires the consent of those persons or organizations (see chapter 1).
- If you have submitted your research to an ethics committee, you must mention this in the report.

Data reporting

- Reporting the frequencies in percentages rather than in exact numbers makes it easier to understand. For example, the following phrase is a typical way for reporting detailed and comprehensive data: "The survey shows that 20 percent of patients . . ." However, when reporting the results for a small number of participants (100 or fewer), the following form is preferable: "Six of the twelve patients indicate that . . ."

Table 8.3. Example of outlining a report before beginning to write		
Component	Function	Concrete content
Introduction	Inform the reader about the motives for the research.	*Personal*: senior year project, interest in treating teenage depression *Professional*: new structure for financing and organizing depression care for youth *Organizational*: changes in care as a result of new policy regarding mental health services for youth
	Inform the reader about the context of the research.	Small, nonprofit community mental health organization Many part-time workers as well as self-employed professionals Many recent organizational developments Current youth mental health policy Relevance for the organization

- Do not present all of your data in the report; use excerpts and summaries instead. Use appendices to provide more extensive material and properly reference this in the text. A reference example is: "See appendix X for a complete overview of the survey results."
- To enhance the credibility and readability of the report, include quotations or other examples from your data. Examples can also serve to concretize or illustrate conclusions.

Distinguish between analysis results, conclusions, reflection, and discussion points

- Conclusions are reached based on the data analysis presented earlier in the report. The reader should, in effect, be able to reach the same conclusions that you provide in the report, based on the data. Substantiate your conclusions with the most important and central findings of your study.
- Do not present new information in the conclusion.
- In the discussion section, you may include your personal opinions and reflections on the research project, particularly as related to your motivation for conducting the research. You should clearly identify your points of view as personal opinions rather than conclusions drawn from the data.

Language

- Use short and powerful statements in straightforward and unambiguous language that is appropriate for the target audience. Instead of saying, "It may be possible that the adolescents felt inadequately treated in the interaction with the activity coordinator," say, "The results suggest that the adolescents were not satisfied with how the activity coordinator treated them."
- However, do not oversimplify, and use proper written language rather than spoken vernacular. Avoid phrasing such as "Training made the nurses better." Instead say, "As a result of the training, nursing staff were more competent when performing patient intake interviews."
- Explain terminology that may not be understood by the reader.

Graphics

- We live in a society that has become increasingly visually oriented. Graphs, tables, charts, images, or cartoons can be more effective in communicating your message than text alone.
- Use self-explanatory labels and titles for these graphics, making their meaning obvious to people who have not yet read the entire text. Information visualized in this manner is given more weight and often stays with the audience longer.
- It is advisable that you only use graphics to convey important research findings (Van der Donk et al., 2014). However, function remains more important than form, and graphics should not draw attention away from the actual content.

Example. Both male and female nursing staff experienced low levels of work-related stress at the beginning of the year. Pressure at work rose strongly for male nurses from January through April, while only some of the female nurses experienced a similar rise in the same time frame. A high peak (in October) is noted for both male and female nursing staff. The most significant divergence in perceived work-related stress between male and female nurses occurred in early May.

A visual presentation of this information adds value to the text and more quickly gets the point across to the reader (figure 8.2).

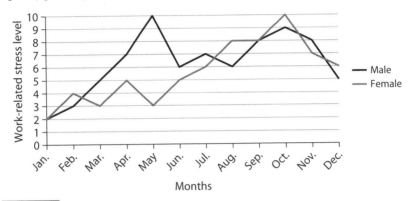

Figure 8.2

Perceived work-related stress (on a scale of 1 to 10) for both male and female nursing staff in 2016

Communication and reflection

- Ask your colleagues to review and comment on the report before you disseminate it to a larger group. Their feedback may enable you to further polish your report and align it with the target audience.

Presentation

Depending on the target audience, you can choose different forms of presentation for disseminating your research results. Make sure you align the presentation form with your selected communication strategy. A large-scale presentation—such as a workshop series or lectures—may not be as useful as a more intimate discussion where the stakeholders are directly involved. Consider an active role in the presentation for colleagues or clients/patients who were involved in the research as a way of reinforcing their ownership of the results.

First Things First

It is understandable that you want to tell the world everything that you learned during the research project. However, this rarely is the best course of action. Information overload may lead to the audience not remembering anything you presented, and it will reduce their capacity to discern your most important conclusions. Presenting only the main research findings generally leads to a better outcome. Hand out the entire research report, or a summary, to interested parties after your presentation.

Involvement

The purpose of the presentation is to generate enthusiasm and to motivate colleagues, clients/patients, and external parties to put your research results into practice. Therefore, your presentation must be in line with the everyday (professional) life, interests, and needs of these groups. Establish a clear link between the research results and daily practice. Familiarize colleagues and other stakeholders with the research results through active participation and let them experiment with the tools, methods, and other instruments that you developed both during and as a result of the research.

A workshop is a good place for actively involving target audiences in discussions and getting their feedback on the products that you developed. You can also use the following forms of presentation during earlier stages or at the end of the research process:

Panelboards, posters, or screens. Place temporary displays or frames with descriptions or graphics about important research results in the lobby, staff room, meeting room, or therapy room. Optionally, you can position yourself near the poster at regular times to answer questions. Display the research results on (interactive) screens in areas within the organization (the cafeteria, for instance) to engage people and stimulate their curiosity about your findings.

Public defense. Ask a select number of people to read the research report prior to your presentation. Invite them to ask critical questions following your presentation before a larger audience. Afterward, distribute copies of the report to interested members.

Speakers' corner. At set times, discuss research issues with interested parties in a designated area or room.

Catchphrases. Display captivating phrases about your research results at highly frequented locations in the organization. For instance: "Did you know ... that 20 percent of staff in our employment program display burnout symptoms? Read all about it in the research report on our website."

Website. Present the research findings on the organization's website and invite colleagues, clients/patients, and other stakeholders to review the results and provide feedback.

Video log, or vlog. Keep people informed by sharing short and inspiring video productions to get them involved in your (preliminary) research findings.

Role-playing. Organize role-plays to clarify important research findings.

Graphic representation. Represent significant findings in the form of a comic book, photo album, (short) animation, or the like.

Quizzes. Compose questions about the research results and organize a quiz.

Panel discussion. Organize a session where panel members discuss statements relating to the research.

Fictional case studies. Organize a group session to discuss a fictional case with links to your most significant research findings.

Seminars. Organize presentations and discussions to inform and engage participants regarding your research project.

Informal exchange. Share the research results with interested parties over lunch, drinks, or a walking meeting.

Flyers and brochures. Draw in colleagues with informative brochures placed in their mailboxes or send digital flyers via email.

Consultation. Visit colleagues, the board, clients/patients, and/or other professional groups to discuss the research results. These consultations can be initiated by you or any of the interested parties.

Lunch meetings. Inform colleagues about your research findings during the lunch break. Alternatively, provide or display additional information for interested parties to review in the break room.

Assessments. Distribute assessment results from your research to provide colleagues with insight into their actions and behavior, as documented in your study. Refer colleagues to your research report for additional information. Ask colleagues to fill out a questionnaire that you used in your research before they read the recommendations in your report.

Prediction. Colleagues project their assumptions about your research results in a questionnaire or during a discussion. For example, health care staff are given a satisfaction survey that was filled out by patients in your study, and the staff are asked to predict the results for each of the questions. Afterward, you present the actual research results.

Roundtable discussions. You and other researchers are each assigned a table. Interested parties can alternate between tables to learn about the research results in informational sessions or discussion rounds.

Exercise 2. Disseminating Research Results (see page 249)

8.4. Implementation

Implementation is described as a systematic process to translate and apply research findings into effective interventions mostly within the context of an organization. Therefore, it is critical to consider relevant decisions needed to adopt the interventions and make necessary adaptions to them so they can be sustained (Damschroder et al., 2009).

Broadly speaking, the two implementation approaches that can be distinguished are the rational model and the participatory model (Grol et al., 2013). In the *rational model*, dissemination starts once the results of the research are known. The research results are translated into new products for the professional practice or into guidelines that are subsequently implemented within the organization.

Example 1. Based on research results, the board of an in-patient treatment clinic decides to implement changes to the safety protocols for its personnel.

Example 2. As part of their degree program, several youth advocates investigated the possibilities for enhancing parents' involvement at a youth detention center. The detention center incorporated the recommendations into its guidelines for daily practice to bring about greater parent involvement.

Within the *participatory model*, both dissemination and implementation take place during the research project. Innovation (change) is implemented in stages in collaboration with stakeholders. The research focuses on designing, testing, and implementing changes in the professional practice. Design research is based on this approach (see chapter 7).

Example. In the context of research regarding the professionalization of educators working at a preschool learning center, a self-assessment instrument has been developed and tested in consultation with the stakeholders. The center will use the instrument for reflecting on its annual performance review meetings.

Stakeholders are often actively involved in practitioner research. Their contribution may result in incremental changes to the design of the study and the results.

Example. As the director of a senior care facility, you are conducting a study to assess the hobbies and social interests of residents. You ask the residents to document their daily activities for one week and to note down any activities that they did not (but would have liked to) engage in on any given day. The research is of great interest to the activity coordinators at the care facility, and the residents frequently share their log entries with them. The activity coordinators realize that a significant number of the residents would like to engage in more music-related activities. Even before the research project is concluded, more such activities are planned to accommodate this desire.

Characteristics of Change

Several characteristics of change that may influence the implementation process are as follows (based on Fullan, 2001; Greenhalgh et al., 2004):

Added Value

Other professionals need to feel that the changes you propose in your research report will effectively make work processes simpler, less costly, or more efficient. If that is the case, change will be perceived as a solution to the practice problem.

Alignment

Changes that are explicitly in line with the values, norms, and vision of your fellow health care and social work professionals, as well as the organization as a whole, will have a better chance of success. If you propose profound deviations from established practices, you will likely encounter stronger resistance—even if your research shows that those changes are required. However, resistance to change need not necessarily stop you from disseminating your findings.

Complexity

The complexity of the changes depends on the scope, the number of people or groups involved, and the degree of change related to the current situation. The more complex the changes, the more intense the effort required to initiate the transformation within the organization. For that reason, it is important that you clarify the overall feasibility of implementing changes and the expected impact of the changes on the organization before disseminating your results. Concurrent implementation of more than one major change will increase the overall complexity of the plan.

Observability

Observability relates to the opportunity for your colleagues to experience or witness examples of the changes in action. Take this into account when planning your research and purposefully involve those individuals or groups that are directly impacted by your research and its results.

> *Example.* The results of your research are outlined in a proposal that aims to stimulate patient involvement in care. However, you have not yet developed supporting material, such as a booklet or training manual. This minimizes the chance of actual change being realized within the organization.

Flexibility and Room to Experiment

The chance of success will be higher when the intended users are given the opportunity to test the proposed changes. Fostering a sense of control over the implementation process among the stakeholders creates a sense of co-ownership and responsibility. Furthermore, support for the changes increases and the new methods or procedures will more likely be adapted to the stakeholders' individual circumstances.

Acceptance through Quality and Clarity

Fellow professionals will adopt the research results if they feel that your research is solid and well founded. Using clear and concrete language in the context of a well-prepared presentation will also increase the likelihood of the research results being applied to the professional practice of your colleagues. Link your new findings and insights to everyday professional situations in order to make the results relatable and acceptable for fellow professionals.

Exercise 3. Characteristics of Change (see page 250)

Stages of Change

When faced with new ideas, people generally go through several stages—orientation, insight, acceptance, change, and maintenance—and the pace at which they do this varies per individual or team (Grol et al., 2013).

Orientation: A need or call for change emerges or is recognized.

Insight: Existing methods and routines are discussed and analyzed along with new possibilities and ways of thinking. Ideas about solutions gradually emerge with a growing sense of confidence that such ideas may address the practice problem and improve the situation. Moving from this stage to the next one depends on whether the stakeholders have developed a clear image of change or not.

Acceptance: In this phase, the intent for practical change becomes concrete. Stakeholders are open, for instance, to different techniques for dialogue, innovative technologies, or new protocols.

Change: New methods and practices are implemented, while old habits and routines are abandoned.

Maintenance: The changes are embedded in the work methods and routine of the everyday professional practice and become an integral part of the organization's quality assurance system.

Resistance to Change

Occasionally, several individuals or groups among the target audience may not accept your research results or your proposed changes.

Example. Medical assistants and nursing staff working in a nursing home have duties and responsibilities that overlap in some areas. The director of the home conducts a study to clarify the problem by mapping the care duties performed by each group. The research leads to the identification of numerous functions that have not been specified in the employees' job descriptions. Those functions are grounded in the everyday professional reality at the nursing home, but they have not been considered as being part of any of the health care providers' jobs. As a result, the medical assistants often perform many of the nursing duties, even though they are not officially expected to do so. The board decides to address the problem by not letting the medical assistants perform nursing duties any longer. The medical assistants oppose the plan, as they fear the changes will partially remove a vital and appealing part of their job.

This entire book is guided by the notion that stakeholders are more likely to embrace and implement the changes that you propose if they are involved in your research from the very beginning. The following section lists several helpful strategies for change implementation.

Implementation Strategies

Practitioner research is typically about increasing stakeholders' involvement in research and effectively working with them to improve the situation by implementing the results. At some stage, your practitioner research concludes while the implementation and integration of your research results continue (Smeijsters et al., 2011). Depending on your position within the organization, the scope of your research results, and practical issues such as time constraints and financial means, you may or may not be responsible for the implementation process. It is advisable that you share with others the implementation responsibilities for projects that have large organizational consequences. You can recommend or apply several different implementation strategies (based on Davis & Taylor-Vaisey, 1997; Grol et al., 2013; Powel et al., 2019):

Education

An educational strategy aims to change the mind-sets and actions of health care and social work professionals and to enhance their competencies (knowledge, skills, and attitudes). This can be achieved through instructional materials (such as videos, manuals, and specialist memorandums), conference presentations, courses, e-learning modules, small-scale training sessions, discussions at team meetings, or guest lectures and trainings from outside experts. Educational strategies can be either optional (voluntary enrollment) or mandatory. It is a major incentive if you are able to offer continuing education credits recognized by the licensing boards of the professionals involved.

Feedback and Reminders

Familiarity with change motivates people to move toward the desired behavior. Examples are goal-oriented coaching, flowcharts and checklists for daily tasks, feedback in teams, focused reflection, and adding new categories and instructions to documentation software.

Organizational and Financial Incentives

Program managers or supervisors can introduce organizational (or financial) incentives to stimulate or enforce the recommended changes. These incentives can include rewriting job descriptions to include the changes, hiring new staff to perform the changes, emphasizing merit-based assessment of performance and input as related to the changes, allocating new funding for the changes, adjusting budgets to account for the changes, or allowing staff to adjust their schedules so as to be able to perform the changes.

Marketing

This strategy focuses on promoting change by influencing opinion. A positive image among staff of the proposed change, and especially having personal experience of benefits resulting from the change, leads to a swifter and smoother implementation. Promoting change can be accomplished by showcasing positive examples from practice, providing user-friendly and appealing training materials, or presenting research results that give an indication of the positive effects that the changes will produce.

Social Interaction

Your colleagues may be motivated to act when they witness positive changes in their fellow professionals or clients/patients, or when they are exposed to inquiries and information about the innovation. That is, the change is not imposed from above but rather inspired by the professional practice of others as communicated by word of mouth. You can stimulate this process by organizing hands-on pilot sessions for new methods or techniques, peer-consultation sessions, or by providing a platform for clients/patients who are requesting change.

Example. A team leader encourages his social workers to be more self-directed in their practice. His practitioner research shows that social workers are open to the idea of self-direction but lack examples. The team leader facilitates the members of the team in developing a plan to support clients in being more self-directed. The plan is implemented. Through this experience, the social workers learn how to translate self-direction into their individual professional lives.

Mandate and Oversight

This strategy comes into play when change in professional practice is mandated from above (federal or state regulations, organizational policy, etc.). Oversight to ensure the implementation of the mandate can accelerate the adoption. Examples include accreditation and licensure requirements, inspection procedures, or contracts with payers/funders.

Exercise 4. Implementation Strategies (see page 250)

8.5. Evaluation

After the conclusion of your research project, you may want to document your new ideas, discussion points, new research questions, and recommendations for future research. You also need to consider innovative ways for tracking important data that help you evaluate the quality of your study's implementation and its success in achieving your stated objectives.

Outlook research inevitably leads to new questions. Record these questions and incorporate them into your research report to document which of these you did not answer in your study and may want to consider in the future.

Integrate your personal opinions, ideas, discussion points, and the significance of the findings for professional practice into your report as well. These ideas and views may be equally important to the readers and provide them with new insights for future research projects.

If the research has led to an innovation, describe how your colleagues can plan for a successful implementation.

Evaluation and Assessment of Practitioner Research

Through conducting your research, you attain invaluable insight and experience. Do your best to write this down in a logbook or journal. These notes can be used to evaluate the research process. Give special attention to those factors or events that helped or hindered your project. Make sure to identify the limitations of your research.

Assessment Criteria

Once your practitioner research concludes, you can perform a personal assessment of the research by answering the following two questions:

1. Was my research successful?
2. What criteria have I used to judge the success of my research?

To help you answer the questions, there are seven assessment criteria to consider. The research project as well as the motives of your colleagues, the board, and/or your study program determine which of these criteria are the most significant. Many of them are interrelated and must be assessed as a whole.

1. *The practitioner research has led to personal development.* This can be gauged in several different ways:
   - You acquired knowledge and new insights on the topic of the research, contributing to your professional development. For example, you now know more about the client/patient population or recent policy developments in the organization in which you work.
   - You developed research skills and an inquisitive mind-set.
   - You experienced personal development in terms of your values and worldview.

   The extent of your personal development as a result of the research is an expression of the *catalytic validity* of the research (Anderson et al., 2007; Herr & Anderson, 2015).

2. *The practitioner research has led to collective development.* The same transformation seen at the personal level for you may have also taken place for others involved in the research. This is called *collective development*. New knowledge and insights, development of research skills, or changes in values can all occur at this level as well. Practitioner research may lead to further development for the members of a multidisciplinary team, for a specific group of professionals, or for the entire staff. In doing so, practitioner research contributes to a learning organization. Collective development is a further expression of the catalytic validity of the research (Anderson et al., 2007; Herr & Anderson, 2015).

3. *The Practitioner Research Method was followed.* The way in which you conducted your practitioner research may constitute an important criterion in the evaluation and assessment of your practitioner research outcomes. One important criterion is whether the relevant key components were completed at least once according to the guidelines described in this book. Another criterion is whether the various key components form a coherent whole. This is part of what is called *process validity* (Anderson et al., 2007; Herr & Anderson, 2015).

4. *The practitioner research project was carried out transparently.* The objective of your research report is to inform others clearly about the methods you used and the knowledge you gained in the process. Writing the research report, communicating the results, and producing additional material for practice (articles, manuals, etc.) are all part of the research and learning process. The degree of transparency you achieved is a further component of process validity (Anderson et al., 2007; Herr & Anderson, 2015).

5. *The practitioner research project was carried out in line with the context.* Context is a great influencing factor in practitioner research as the goal is to solve everyday problems in a specific setting. The degree to which your research is in line with this setting is a criterion when evaluating the research. This is yet another part of process validity (Anderson et al., 2007; Herr & Anderson, 2015) and takes into account the following:

   - Whether the practice problem was defined in a way to be relevant for the setting.

   - The degree to which the specific characteristics of the setting were taken into account when executing the research activities.

   - The degree to which the research results are relevant for both the setting and the specific target audience.

6. *The practitioner research project has contributed to the solution of the practice problem.* The objective of practitioner research is to contribute to solving a practice problem. The research question indicates which part of the practice problem your research addressed. The extent to which the research solved the practice problem is a measure of success. This criterion addresses the *outcome validity* of your research (Anderson et al., 2007; Herr & Anderson, 2015).

7. *The practitioner research project was carried out in participation with others.* Third parties play an active role throughout the practitioner research process. The extent of others' involvement affects the chances of your research results being used in practice and thus leading to real change. This criterion addresses the *democratic validity* and *dialogic validity* of the research (Anderson et al., 2007; Herr & Anderson, 2015).

Exercise 5. Evaluation and Assessment (see page 250)

8.6. Summary

This chapter explained how to document and present your research results and how to implement changes based on those results. Documentation and implementation is the final component of the research cycle, but it needs to be taken into account throughout the research process. You must continually involve stakeholders from professional practice settings in your research in order to facilitate the dissemination and implementation of your findings. This requires insight into the target audience—those people who are directly impacted by your findings.

You disseminate your research results by documenting and presenting the new knowledge and insights gained. You select the appropriate communication strategy using a communication matrix template. Your research report documents important details about the study to substantiate the methods and results, and documentation can take various forms. The most important components of a research report are the abstract, introduction, problem definition, approach, ethical considerations, findings, conclusion, and discussion.

You take the various interests of the target audience(s) into account when presenting the research. You can choose from several forms of presentation to disseminate your research results within the organization.

Where the research requires changes in professional practice, you not only consider the dissemination of the results but also the most suitable implementation strategy. The rational model and participatory model are two different implementation approaches. Design research is based on the participatory model.

When faced with change, people generally go through several stages. Not all members of the target audience are necessarily in the same stage of change. The characteristics of the proposed changes influence the implementation process.

Both looking back to the past and planning for the future characterize the final stage of research. A systematic evaluation and assessment of the research should take place, focusing on various aspects related to the motives that you or others expressed at the start of your research project.

EXERCISES

Exercise 1. Communication Matrix

This exercise is about identifying documentation and presentation strategies within an organizational context using a communication matrix template.

The communication matrix from section 8.1, based on Van Ruler (1998), provides a helpful framework for planning your documentation and presentation activities. For each of the cells in the communication matrix, write down several forms of documentation and presentation that are acceptable and frequently conducted within the organization. Complement these entries with forms of documentation and presentation that have not yet been used within the organization but that could be utilized in the future.

Exercise 2. Disseminating Research Results

Section 8.4 described various forms of presentation to disseminate your research results. Which form(s) do you think are most appropriate in the following case?

> You work in a department that provides care to Alzheimer patients. You have difficulty finding an approach that enhances the quality of life for terminal dementia patients and you wish to explore this issue. You come across a possible solution in the form of the research-based sense activation method. You decide to explore

how this method can be applied in your professional practice. The research leads to positive results in the lives of Alzheimer patients. Your supervisor wants this method adopted by other practitioners in your department.

Exercise 3. Characteristics of Change

Several characteristics of change increase the likelihood of a successful implementation of recommended changes in an organization (Fullan, 2001; Greenhalgh et al., 2004). These characteristics are added value, alignment, complexity, observability, flexibility and room to experiment, acceptance through quality and clarity.

List a few innovations that were implemented in your professional practice in recent years. Assess and discuss these innovations based on the above characteristics. Optionally, do the same for your own research results.

Exercise 4. Implementation Strategies

Think of an innovation that has recently been implemented in your organization or in an organization with which you are familiar. Go back in time and determine what implementation strategies were used. Try to imagine what other strategies could have been used.

Exercise 5. Evaluation and Assessment

Perform this exercise in collaboration with a group of stakeholders. All participants first answer the following question individually on paper: "What do you think constitutes success regarding this research project?" Share the answers with the group and sort them based on the assessment criteria described in this chapter. Discuss the assessment criteria used by each member of the group and why each chose the criteria they did.

REFERENCES

Altrichter, H., Feldman, A., Posch, P., & Somekh, B. (2008). *Teachers investigate their work: An introduction to action research across the profession*. Routledge.

Anderson, G. L., Herr, K., & Nihlen, A. S. (Eds.). (2007). *Studying your own school: An educator's guide to practitioner action research*. Corwin Press.

Damschroder, L. J., Aron, D. C., Keith, R. E., Kirsh, S. R., Alexander, J. A., & Lowery, J. C. (2009). Fostering implementation of health services research findings into practice: A consolidated framework for advancing implementation science. *Implementation Science, 4*(1), 50.

Davis, D. A., & Taylor-Vaisey, A. (1997). Translating guidelines into practice: A systematic review of theoretic concepts, practical experience and research evidence in the adoption of clinical practice guidelines. *Canadian Medical Association Journal, 157,* 408–416.

Fullan, M. (2001). *The new meaning of educational change*. Teachers College Press.

Greenhalgh, T., Robert, G., Macfarlane, F., Bate, P., & Kyriakidou, O. (2004). Diffusion of innovations in service organizations: Systematic review and recommendations. *Milbank Quarterly, 82*(4), 581–629.

Grol, R., Wensing, M., Eccles, M., & Davis, D. (Eds.). (2013). *Improving patient care: The implementation of change in health care*. John Wiley & Sons.

Hall, G. M. (2013). *How to write a paper*. Wiley-Blackwell.

Herr, K., & Anderson, G. L. (2015). *The action research dissertation: A guide for students and faculty*. (2nd ed.). Sage.

Powell, B. J., et al. (2019). Enhancing the impact of implementation strategies in healthcare: A research agenda. *Frontiers in Public Health*, *7*, 3.

Smeijsters, H., et al. (2011). *Kenmerken, randvoorwaarden en criteria van praktijkgericht zorgonderzoek* [Features, requirements and criteria of practice-based research in health care]. HBORaad, ZonMW.

Van der Donk, C., Van Lanen, B., & Wright, M. T. (2014). *Praxisforschung im Sozial- und Gesundheitswesen* [Practitioner research in social work and health care]. Verlag Hans Huber.

Van Ruler, A. A. (1998). *Strategisch Management van Communicatie: Introductie van het communicatiekruispunt* [Strategic Communication Management: Introducing the communication matrix]. Samson.

World Wide Writing (2019). *Onderzoeksverslag* [Research report]. https://worldwidewriting.ruhosting.nl

Using Sources

G ood practitioner research is informed by the results of previously conducted scientific studies and professional guidelines and standards. Such sources are documented in various formats and can enrich key components of your practitioner research project in different ways:

- During the orientation stage, you begin your literature review and collect practical data to enrich the exploratory problem analysis described in section 2.3, techniques 5 and 8.

- During the focusing stage, you complete your literature review in order to further explore and redefine your practice problem, clarify the scope of your inquiry, and conceptualize a framework for your research using current theories and models.

- During the data collection stage, relevant findings from scientific and professional sources will help you answer several of your sub-questions and provide you with the information needed for developing your data collection instruments.

- During the design stage, the principles of your design could be largely validated based on data provided by external and internal sources.

- During the documentation and presentation stage, information collected throughout your review could be used to enhance the quality of your discussion about the meaning and implication of the findings for practice. You may review additional sources to provide more food for thought for your readers or to highlight future steps, questions, and theories that could emerge from the research.

The first part of this appendix provides an overview of different types of textual sources (A.1). The second and third parts cover how to identify suitable sources and how to assess their reliability and significance (A.2 and A.3). Lastly, the standard styles for citing different varieties of sources can be found in the final part (A.4). You can refer to this addendum anytime you need to conduct a literature review.

A.1. Textual Sources

All digital and paper-based sources can be categorized into *public sources* and *internal sources*.

Public Sources

Public sources can be further classified into two types: (1) peer-reviewed sources found in journals, books, databases, websites of professional organizations, and so on; and (2) non-peer-reviewed sources containing studies or reports from a single organization and anecdotal evidence (also called *gray literature*). Gray literature can be from public, private, nongovernmental, or academic institutions, but it also includes commercial or other types of information found in the popular press. Both peer-reviewed and gray literature can be found in various formats. Peer review of scientific articles is considered a standard quality procedure within the academic community and is meant to improve the quality of (written) material through critical review and feedback by fellow professionals who work in the same areas of research.

Sources for Specialized Literature and Studies

Specialized literature can be found in books, articles, and research reports published on almost every topic from various disciplinary, professional, and technical backgrounds, such as psychology, pedagogy, social work, nursing, physical therapy, occupational therapy, medicine, public health, research methods, and so on. Nowadays, such sources are becoming increasingly accessible in digital forms and through online libraries. However, brick-and-mortar libraries are often still the best place for many classic paper-based titles or for people who prefer to read from the hard copies.

Example. John is the chief supervisor of the emergency department of a community hospital. He wishes to assess patient-handoff procedures after release from the emergency department. John's main concern is about the lack of proper communication between members of the health care team in different departments, resulting in potential risks regarding patient care and safety. His main research question is around duties and responsibilities of the team members. He finds the topic of patient handoffs in a few specialized books and articles to better understand the term, potential risks and pitfalls, and the necessary elements of care that could be improved with better coordination and proper procedures. At later stages, John uses the results of his literature review to draft a flowchart and to develop a questionnaire to assess the current status of patient-handoff practices in the hospital.

Policy Documents and Reports

Almost every professional practice institution is set up according to national and local policies and procedures that clarify the administrative, funding, and other relevant aspects of the care in order to ensure quality, proper functioning, and coordination of health and social services. Therefore, conducting practitioner research often requires in-depth knowledge of certain policies and guidelines relevant to the identified practice problem. Such information is often documented in policy papers, textbooks, and special reports. Furthermore, you may find good answers to some of your questions regarding the consequences of budget cuts, accountability measures, interagency partnership and coordination, or changes in the overall budget of health care and social services. Other questions that could be answered with policy documents and reports may be, for example, what are the benefits of e-health for health care and social services? What does the Health Insurance Portability and Accountability Act (HIPPA) entail? And how are costs related to long-term disabilities, home care, and community services coverage?

Newspapers and Magazines

A great amount of useful information related to health and social services can be found in the popular press, such as newspapers and magazines. Some of this information is a popularization of findings from scientific studies or policy statements. Other information may include commentaries from experts, reports of roundtable and panel discussions, anecdotal stories, human interest stories, and news. It is important to review and critically check the credibility of the information from the popular press, as it may represent special interests and could be biased. It is recommended to first critically review the soundness of the investigation method used by the author and the credibility of the sources cited before deciding to include the results in your literature review. It is always advisable to consult the original sources, if possible.

> *Example.* Based on a newspaper article, a social work student concludes that the health of the city's elderly is being negatively affected by cuts to the Meals on Wheels program for seniors.

This is an example of a claim that could bias your research. Since newspapers include various forms of articles—from opinion pieces to news analysis to actual news stories—there is a greater or lesser degree of verification needed depending on what type of article you're referencing. Newspaper articles may provide important insights and raise noteworthy assumptions, but they are generally not sufficient for providing answers to your research question.

Websites and Social Media

With the invention of the internet and social media, an overwhelming amount of information is currently available to us through numerous websites, blogs, and social media platforms. However, since it's possible for any member of the public to publish information on the internet, it is sometimes very difficult to distinguish credible information from false information. For that reason, online sources should be treated with particular caution. If used properly, the internet can be a valuable source for deepening your understanding of the practice problem and planning your research. The following example illustrates a well-considered use of online information and resources.

Example. Sasha is running a music therapy program for children ages 12 to 18 with developmental and learning disabilities. She faces a problem of not being able to fully engage the children and their parents in the activities outside the classroom. Since music therapy was a fairly new concept for these children, Sasha conducted a search over the internet to learn from different music therapy programs. She identified several programs with similar protocols and various innovative approaches. This gave her many ideas about things that she had not considered before. In addition, she found a listserv associated with a credible national organization through which novel evidence-based information on music therapy is distributed. Lastly, she decided to create a social media group with the parents to share news about her program and to further explore opportunities for more active participation of the children and their parents in the activities.

Internal Sources

Internal sources include all materials, including documents and databases, that are only accessible to members of an organization. These materials are produced within the organization, either as part of routine administrative and regulatory procedures or for other purposes related to the professional practice, such as fundraising, evaluation of services, or communication with internal and external stakeholders. Every organization generates a considerable amount of material that could be extremely informative for practitioner research. However, before collecting and using such information you need to carefully assess the sensitivity and confidentiality of the information and to obtain the necessary consent for using the material in your research. A variety of internal sources are listed here.

Organizational Policy Documents

National policies are often translated into operational policies at the organizational level. But also, each organization has its own traditions and operating procedures. Such policies are often documented in various ways, such as in the organization's strategic plan, standard operating procedures, annual reports, specific project reports, client/patient and organizational assessments and surveys, and so on. Such documents provide an important framework for understanding the setting and context of your practitioner research.

Informational Education and Communication Materials

Most organizations develop different kinds of informational education and communication materials in the form of posters, brochures, and pamphlets for communication and educational purposes. In addition, organization websites usually contain basic information, recent news and newsletters, publications, and reports. In practitioner research, it is critical to review such materials to both become aware of current practices and identify high priority areas for research.

Internal Communication and Service Statistics

Every organization produces a significant amount of data in the form of internal communications and service statistics. Such data can be found in meeting notes, interview reports, client/patient records, statistics on referrals, treatment results, and evaluation reports. Some sources may contain confidential information and should be used only with special permission. Some organizations may impose restrictions on the use of confidential or private documents and may not allow using such resources for research and publication purposes.

A.2. Finding the Needed Sources

Extracting the most relevant and worthwhile information from the entire available literature is a Herculean task. Here we provide you with a few guidelines on how to find the most useful sources for your practitioner research study. We recommend that you begin the process by reading a relevant section of a recommended textbook on fundamental aspects of your practice problem. Textbooks are important sources for basic and technical information, often providing a good overview. Every college recommends specialized texts for their respective courses that are considered key publications for both introductory and expert subjects. You may get access to that information through checking the college's website or course syllabi, as well as by consulting a curriculum specialist or someone from an academic bookstore.

Choosing a relevant textbook from a recommended reading list can be a good starting point for conducting your literature review. Such textbooks can then further guide your next steps by providing you with the bibliographical information for other useful sources (e.g., journal articles, reports, case studies) where you can find more detailed information. You can also do this by asking any experts whom you might know (e.g., a former professor, a mentor, or a colleague). In addition to recommended textbooks, you may start reading other key publications related to your subject of interest where an overview of the field have been presented, such as systematic review articles, meta-analysis studies, doctoral dissertations, literature reviews written by senior experts, and statements from professional organizations summarizing current literature and practice. Here we provide you with some ideas about where to find them.

Learning Centers and Libraries

Many organizations have small or large libraries with collections of useful books, journals, magazines, and other sources of information related to their professional practice. Furthermore, some organizations have strategic partnerships and collaborations with other libraries and learning centers where members of one organization can borrow from others. Most colleges and universities have larger libraries with more extensive collections. We suggest that you spend some time to find out about the libraries and learning centers that are available to you. Most libraries offer free access to certain online resources that would otherwise cost you a fee or require a subscription.

Online Sources and Databases

Digital sources have become the easiest and the most convenient way of accessing both scientific literature and publications of professional bodies. However, online searches can result in an overwhelming amount of information that is not relevant or trustworthy. In addition, some published articles and resources are not free of charge. Therefore, many specific databases have been created for archiving relevant literature and making it more accessible by charging a subscription fee. Some libraries pay the subscription fees for certain databases, making them available free of charge for their members (see above). Some databases are more general and can be used for access to abstracts of many published articles. We suggest that after clarifying your search strategies and identifying your keywords (more on this in a minute), you should start with large databases and then explore other specialized databases for more technical resources and to access the full text of materials. Here are a few examples of well-known online databases for published scientific materials in different fields:

Google Scholar provides an easy way to search for scholarly literature from a variety of disciplines. Through Google Scholar, you can simultaneously search multiple sources—such as articles, dissertations, edited volumes and books, reports, policy documents, abstracts from academic publishers and professional societies, and other online repositories.

PubMed contains over 26 million citations for biomedical literature from Medline, life science journals, and online books. Citations may include links to full-text content from PubMed Central and publisher websites.

Scopus is the largest database for abstracts and citations of peer-reviewed literature in scientific journals, books, and conference proceedings. Scopus has made it easy to track, analyze, and visualize research material and resources using novel and smart tools. Scopus provides a comprehensive overview of research and scientific materials in the fields of science, technology, medicine, social sciences, and humanities.

PsycINFO is the most comprehensive index in psychology and other associated fields of science, with over 1.7 million citations and abstracts of journal articles, book chapters and books, technical reports, and dissertations. Its holdings include material from 1,700 periodicals in over 30 languages.

Science Direct provides abstracts and indexing for more than 1,800 journals related to humanities and physical, biological, and social sciences. Full text of more than 800 journals is available and many of them are in languages other than English.

Social Work Abstracts offers extensive coverage of more than five hundred social work and human services journals dating back to 1965. Researchers, students, and practitioners can find scholarly and professional perspectives on subjects such as therapy, education, human services, addictions, child and family welfare, mental health, and civil and legal rights.

CINAHL is an index of English-language and selected other-language journal articles about nursing, allied health, biomedicine and health care.

There are other databases and online resources that contain useful evidence-based materials, online forums, newsgroups, and regular newsletters related to health and social services. These resources are often maintained by government organizations, academic institutions, professional organizations, or panels of experts. Here are examples of well-known sources where you can find useful information and sign up for their services:

United States National Institutes of Health: www.nih.gov

National Association of Social Workers: www.socialworkers.org

American Psychological Association: www.apa.org

American Association of Colleges of Nursing: www.aacnnursing.org

American Occupational Therapy Association: www.aota.org

US Department of Health and Human Services: www.hhs.gov

Agency for Healthcare Research and Quality: www.ahrq.gov

United States Health Information Knowledgebase: https://ushik.ahrq.gov

Medline: www.medline.com

Healthdata.gov

Healthcare.gov

Sources such as SpringerLink and Cochrane Library are only open to license-holding organizations, but many college or university libraries provide free access to them.

Further Tips for Searching Online Sources

There are strategic ways for effectively filtering relevant information so as to avoid finding unrelated materials while searching online. The following tips can help you achieve better results:

- Before conducting the search, create a list of relevant keywords that you want to use.
- Look beyond the first 10 hits and further refine your keywords based on the initial results.
- You can reduce the number of hits by combining your keywords. By using the plus sign (+), you will get only hits that contain all keywords (e.g., repeat + offender + rehabilitation).
- Exact phrasing can be searched by enclosing the keywords in quotation marks (e.g., "Affordable Care Act").
- You can use the term "author" to search for resources written by certain experts.
- Many articles are published in PDF format. You can search specifically for PDF files by using the search command "filetype:pdf" (other file extensions can be found with this command as well, such as "filetype:doc" or "filetype:ppt").

Within relevant materials, there are major variations in terms of the trustworthiness and the significance of the information. Therefore, it is important to assess the usefulness and reliability of the sources before deciding to cite them in your work. Furthermore, in practitioner research you often deal with issues that require exploring sources beyond the scope of the typically cited literature. For example, a policy paper written by the Department of Health and Human Services and a story in the popular press written by a social work professional with 25 years of experience are vastly different sources, yet both may contain valuable information for your research. Therefore, it is important to consider relevant quality control criteria for assessing their usefulness and reliability.

To assess the credibility of sources, you often need to ask the following questions:

To what extent is the information in this source relevant to my research objectives? (relevance)

To what extent can I rely on this source? (reputation)

Has this source been cited by others? (recognition)

Can the information in this source be found in other sources as well? (corroboration)

Linking the Source to the Objective

Is your chosen source relevant to your research objective? Will the source help your research? To make these determinations, explicitly state why you need the information in that source and how exactly the information will inform your inquiry.

Example. Another practitioner researcher study made important observations analyzing the quality and effectiveness of the same worksheets that you are using in your counseling sessions. She has published the results in a practice journal. You might find this study relevant to your objective because the information can help you to apply the findings and to focus on areas that have not been fully analyzed. In addition, you may decide to use and adapt the data collection instrument for your practitioner research study.

Next, critically assess how applicable the source of the information is to the context of your research.

Example. You are a psychotherapist using drama therapy for a group of young clients dealing with anxiety and depression. Your research intends to assess the feasibility, acceptability, and effectiveness of semi-structured assignments that could foster more creativity and participant involvement in the process. You come across a recently published report from a panel of drama therapy experts. After examining the report, you realize it is about assessing the effectiveness of assignments that are more structured than the ones you intend to use, but you still might want to learn about some of the core elements that make the assignments effective. Obviously, the report is not fully applicable, but you can note its specific areas of applicability to your research, and those findings can help you identify the gaps as well as the need for including additional sources that discuss less-structured assignments.

Consider the feasibility and practicality of the tools and methods within the context of your professional practice.

Example. You are a public health educator conducting practitioner research in one of the inner-city high schools of Baltimore, Maryland, that has high dropout rates compared to the city average. You intend to evaluate a contingency management program by rewarding good academic and interpersonal behaviors. You believe that having a reward system would help the students improve their academic performance as well as the quality of social interactions between peers. However, your program uses an exact replica of an evidence-based program conducted in Chicago inner-city schools. You come across a systematic review article published in the *American Journal of Public Health* in which 65 different school-based incentive programs—including the one that you are using—are discussed and compared. In this case, your source can help you identify alternatives to the program in Chicago, examining the strengths and weaknesses of each program. On that basis, you can consider how best to adapt your program by incorporating novel aspects of other initiatives.

Critically review internal policy documents and sources by considering their relevance, currency, and significance.

Example. You are a nursing student doing your internship in a local community health center in a low-income inner-city neighborhood of Cleveland, Ohio. You are tasked with reviewing the quality aspects of a patient-education program aimed at reducing the readmission rates of those treated for cardiovascular diseases. After reviewing a commentary from a health care organization leader, you realize that the success of a patient education program depends on the involvement of other family members and community health workers. So you decide to review internal documents and reports related to the organization's past experiences and policies related to family-oriented educational programs using community health workers. However, you determine that many of the reports are too old to be included, and some policy documents are on similar topics but are not quite relevant to your subject of interest. Finally, based on a recommendation from a senior practitioner, you learn about a specific task force that worked for a few months on this topic. You make a request and are granted permission to review meeting notes and reports prepared by the task force. In this case, such information could be highly relevant to your needs and significantly enrich your research.

Assessing Source Reliability

To assess the reliability of your sources, use the following sets of questions and their respective quality criteria:

1. Who is the publisher of the textual source? Is your source published by a credible publisher or institution? Has the publisher received high reviews for producing quality materials? Is it peer-reviewed? What is the journal's impact factor?*

2. Who has validated, endorsed, listed, and used the textual source? Has it been recommended for any courses or training workshops? Is it listed among recommended resources of information by senior experts or institutions? What do previous readers and reviewers say about the source? What are some of the strengths and weaknesses mentioned by the readers and reviewers?

3. What is the ranking or level of attention given to the textual source? Is it known for providing a set of recommendations by a group of experts? Is it known for providing mandatory guidelines for professional practice? Is the material or manuscript cited often?

4. Is the information provided by the source verifiable? Does it include facts and statistics (e.g., US unemployment rates) that could be verified by searching the original sources? Does it include detailed information about their investigational methods? If applicable, what kind of research methodologies have they been using (e.g., systematic review, cross-sectional, case-control, clinical trial)? Have the authors made a compelling argument about handling different potential biases and confounders? Are the results confirmed by other relevant studies?

5. Who is the author or the team of authors of the title? What is the disciplinary perspective and level of seniority of the author or the team of authors? What are the organizational backgrounds of the authors? Have the all the authors published other relevant high-impact materials? Has their previous work received favorable reviews from readers?†

6. What is the quality of the writing and the logical flow of the argument? How convincing is the argument? How extensive is the authors' knowledge of previous research presented in the introduction and the discussion? What did the authors base their conclusions on and is it convincing? Are the references used for the material properly cited according to a standard style? (See section A.4 for more information.)

---

* An impact factor is a quality measure for peer-reviewed journals reflecting the average annual number of citations to articles published in that journal. For example, an impact factor of 3 means on average recent papers published by the journal have received three citations in the subsequent year. In general, journals with higher impact factors are considered more credible.

† Author and coauthor background is important because it contributes to the author's unique perspective and approach that they might have on a particular topic. For example, a policy officer at an insurance company will have a different point of view from a member of the House of Representatives or the director of a care facility. Similarly, the disciplinary perspective of a psychology professor could be vastly different from that of a nursing professor.

To assess the reliability of other sources of information—such as published popular press interviews and stories, online discussions and blogs, meeting notes and other internal documents, presentations at conferences and seminars, and so on—there are other relevant quality standard questions that you can ask, including:

- What are the primary sources of information?
- Is the information provided considered facts or expert opinions?
- Are the presented facts verifiable through other sources?
- Is there general agreement regarding expert opinions presented by the source or is there controversy?
- What are the main arguments presented by the proponents and opponents about the experts' opinion?
- Are internal documents properly organized, dated, and recorded?
- Did any of the discussion result in decisions and actions related to your practitioner research?
- What information was used to make decisions?
- Is there any information that you can use to verify the implementation of the decisions and their results?

A.4. Referencing and Citation

A bibliography is usually included in research plans, reports, and articles and is often included at the very end of each. The bibliography lists all the sources that were used to gather the information included in a final research document. You need to refer to your sources according to a standard style anytime you use any of the information in your research. This includes information said or written by another person, even if you paraphrase the information in your own words. This is necessary both to give credit to those who have produced the materials and to enable your readers to verify your statements by consulting your sources for more details. Lack of proper referencing of information could be considered plagiarism, which has serious ramifications for a researcher's reputation. Usually you cite the sources as abbreviated text or by using a numeric note system in the body of your text, and your readers find the complete bibliographical information at the end of the document or the end of each chapter.

To facilitate traceability and ensure uniformity of bibliographical references, several standard referencing styles have been invented. Citation styles mainly differ based on the location, order, and syntax of the information for different types of sources. Some commonly used referencing styles are the Modern Language Association (MLA), American Psychological Association (APA), Chicago Manual of Style, Harvard style, and Vancouver style. Prior to writing your reports for educational or publication purposes, make sure that you follow the referencing style prescribed by the publication (or your instructor). If no styles are recommended, make sure that you consistently follow one of the standard styles of your choosing. Do not combine different styles of referencing in one document. Here we present APA style with examples from the *Publication Manual of the American Psychological Association* (7th ed., 2020).

You can learn about the other styles online. Also, there are software programs such as EndNote and Reference Manager that can help create citations and automatically change the format to another style when needed.

In-Text Citation of Sources

You need to specify your sources when you are basing your argument on ideas or information provided by other authors (or from your own previously published work). In some reports, authors may choose to include the entire reference in the body of the text or place it in a footnote on the same page. However, in most cases, abbreviated versions of the sources are cited in the text and refer to a list of references with complete citation information at the end of a chapter or the end of the full article or book. Full citations include authors' names, the title and date of the publication, the publishing entity, and other details (e.g., volume, page number, other specific identifying numbers). In the APA format, in-text citations include the name of up to two authors and the year of publication (separated by a comma), and they appear following the relevant information in the body text.

> *Example.* Tailored care is a form of health care or social assistance treatment approach that is designed based on the needs of individual patients (Wan, 2018).

When referring to several sources at the same time, you must list them all—in alphabetical order by each first author's last name followed by date of the publication—in one set of parentheses (separated by semicolons) after the information being cited.

> *Example.* The main focus in the process of providing health care is shifting from solely responding to existing limitations to reflecting on opportunities for improving health outcomes (Andermann, 2016; Boyce & Brown, 2019; Daniel et al., 2018).

If you decide to use the name of an author as part of the narrative in the body of the text, you can just include the year of publication in parentheses:

In this context, Wan (2018) described the principles of the tailored care concept.

Chakrabarti (2014) has provided a different definition of treatment compliance.

To improve readability, shorten those references coauthored by more than two authors by listing the full name of the first author followed by the Latin abbreviation "et al." (*et alii*, "and others"):

There are different interpretations about the effects of market and economic forces on health care and social work practices (Daniel et al., 2018).

According to Daniel et al. (2018), there are different interpretations about the effects of market and economic forces on health care and social work practices.

The names of the additional authors will be mentioned in the bibliography upon first use. Note, however, that from the second reference onward, the abbreviation "et al." may be used again instead. The exception is when the source has more than five authors; these may be indicated with "et al." from the first time the source is referenced in the bibliography.

Literal or direct quotations in the body of the text are referred to by author, year of publication, and the page number of the original text. If the quotation is entirely printed on one page, use the abbreviation "p." for the page (e.g., p. 16). If the quotation is from multiple pages, use "pp." (e.g., pp. 16–18). Cite quotations when the information cannot be rephrased, for instance when using definitions or particularly poignant statements. Enclose direct quotations with double quotation marks.

Example. "Tailored care implies that the needs and specific characteristics of patients are taken into account when providing care," says Wan (2018, p. 4).

Bibliographical Structure

In the APA bibliography style, references are listed alphabetically by the last name of the first author to make it easy for readers to find the reference they need.

Multiple sources by the same author(s) will be listed in chronological order, with the oldest publication first and most recent publication last.

Below are a few examples of how to cite different kinds of references using APA style.

Books

Author's last name, Initials. (Year). *Title: Subtitle* (when appropriate). Publisher.

Single author:

Stuart, C. (2009). *Foundations of child and youth care.* Kendall Hunt.

Thompson, N. (2005). *Understanding social work: Preparing for practice.* Palgrave Macmillan.

Multiple authors:

Weisz, J., & Kazdin, A. (2017). *Evidence-based psychotherapies for children and adolescents.* Guildford Press.

Organizational authors:

American Psychiatric Association. (2013). *Diagnostic and statistical manual of mental disorders.* American Psychiatric Publishing.

Manuals, Magazines, and Newspapers

The rules are slightly different when referencing manuals, magazines, or newspapers.

Online magazine article:

Author's last name, Initials. (Year, Month Day). Title of the article. *Title of the Magazine.* URL

Ducharme, J. (2020, February 12). Juul advertised its products on kids' websites, new lawsuit alleges. *Time*. https://time.com/5783022/juul-kids-advertising

Print magazine article:

Author's last name, Initials. (Year, Month Day). Title of the article. *Title of the Magazine, volume*(issue), pages.

Newspaper article:

Author's last name, Initials. (Year, Month Day). Title of the article. *Title of the Newspaper*. URL (if applicable)

Journal Articles

Author's last name, Initials. (Year). Title of the article. *Journal Title, volume*(issue), pages. DOI or URL (if available)

Levinger, M., & Segev, E. (2018). Admission and completion of social work programs: Who drops out and who finishes? *Journal of Social Work, 18*(1), 23–45. https://doi.org/10.1177/1468017316651998

Online Resources

Webpage:

Author, Initials. (Year). Webpage/Article title. Website (omit if it is listed as author). URL

Centers for Disease Control and Prevention. (2020). Addressing health and educational disparities. https://www.cdc.gov/healthyyouth/disparities/action.htm

Whole website reference:

Do not create references or in-text citations for whole websites; instead, provide the name of the website in the running text and include the URL in parentheses.

If no date is listed for any type of source, indicate this by using the abbreviation "n.d." (no date).

Centers for Disease Control and Prevention (CDC). (n.d.). *Understanding evidence: Evidence based decision-making summary*. Retrieved March 1, 2021. https://vetoviolence.cdc.gov/apps/evidence/docs/EBDM_82412.pdf.

Index

Page numbers in **boldface** indicate figures and tables.

Excel, 111, 178, 181–182, 197

exit interviews, 11, 95, 142

exit survey, 99

experiential learning, 7, **7**

expert systems, 219

exploratory problem analysis, 48, 49, 59, 60, 211, 253

exploratory research, 53, 208, 210, 211, 220

expressive data collection, 102, 159–161

face-to-face interviews, 101

feasibility (of implementing changes), 212, 243

filter (or contingency) questions, 154–155

findings, research, 4, 10, 16, 20, 65, 177, 234, 238, 240, 241

flexibility, 102, 109, 159, 243, 250

flowcharts, 51, **51**, 245

flyers, 241

focal points (for document analysis), 122, 127; closed-option, 128; numerical, 128; open-ended (qualitative), 127–129; scaled, 128

focus group, 95, 99, 142, 223

formative evaluation, 225, 227

freewriting, 52, 218

frequencies (totals), calculating, 182

frequency and severity of practice problems, 66, 67

funding, 12, 22, 25, 33, 42, 87, 112, 115, 245, 254

Gantt chart, 111, 115, 117

GNU PSPP, 178, 181, 197

graphic representation, 240

graphics, 238, 240

group discussions, 61, 93, 102, 142, 159, 201

guidelines for documenting systematic observation, 134

guidelines in achieving validity and reliability, 20

health care settings, 26

Health Insurance Portability and Accountability Act (HIPAA), 31

health professional, 2

hidden observation, 130, 133

human participants, 110

human subjects research, 30

idea advocate, 221

images, 160, 197, 205, 238

implementation, 241–242

implementation science, 5, 31

implementation stage, 8

implementation strategies, viii, 230, 245–249

incentive, 20, 26, 31, 109, 245

incentives, organizational and financial, 245

in-depth interview, 69, 93, 100, 101, 118,

in-depth problem analysis, viii, 64, 65, 89, 211

individual interviews, 94, 95, 118, 142, 190

inductive process, 188

inferential statistics, 6, 178

informational material, 75, 79, 218

information bias, 20

information overload, 75, 79, 218, 239,

informed consent, 30, 100, 148, 172, 236

innovation, 3, 242, 246

Innovation Loop, ix, 11, **11**, 13, 15, 31, **207**, 207–208, **217**, 217–227

inquisitive mind-set, 3, 31, 83, 247

institutional ethics committee (IEC), 30

institutional review board (IRB), 30, 35

instrument, stability of, 19

intentional observations, 3

internal sources, 46, 97, 253–256

intersubjectivity, 133

interval variable, 179–182, 186, 188; analysis methods, 180–188

intervention, 208, 227

intervention assimilation, 225

intervention bias, 20

intervention research, 5–6; intervention development and testing / documentation and presentation, 110; intervention group, 100

interventions, 2, 208–210, **211**, 227; minor interventions, 209; modifications to existing interventions, 210; novel interventions, 210

research strategy, 115. *See also* research objectives; research questions; research unit

research unit, 105

resistance to change, 244

retrospective data, 97

return on investment, 29

revise and validate, 101

risks, 30

role-playing, 102, 158–160, 240

roundtable discussions, 241

safety, 165

sample, 106, 178; convenience sampling 107; purposive sampling, 108; random or probability sampling, 106–107; representative sample, 106, 116; reputational sampling, 108; snowball sampling, 106

scientific discoveries, 31

scorecards, 103, 163

secondary data, 97, 176

selection bias, 20

self-assessment instrument, 242

self-direction, 245–246

self-reflection, 116

self-reflective report, 45

site visits, 104–105, 166–167

small-scale testing, 223

snowball sampling, 107

social desirability bias, 20

social experiments, 102, 103, 164–165

social interaction, 246

social mapping, 233

social networks, 26, 32

social service settings, 25–28

solutions and improvement strategies for practice problems, 67

speakers' corner, 240

speech bubbles, 161

SPSS, 178, 181–182

stages of change, 244

stakeholders, 9, 17, 21–22, 46, 59–61, 72, 116–117, 211–214, 217, 221

standard deviation, 181

standardized tests, 99, 156; data analysis for 187–188, 219

statistics, 178; descriptive statistics, 178; inferential statistics, 6, 176, 178

stigmatization, 30

story dialogue, 162

storytelling, 102, 162

strategic approach, 28

strategic needs, 29

subjective answers, 101

sub-questions, 95, 176, 212, 236

summative (final) evaluation, 225, 227

surveying, 99, 101, 102, 151–155, 159; refining and validating questionnaires, 153–155, 156; selecting or developing survey instruments, 152–153

SurveyMonkey, 151

surveys, 95, 100

systematic observation, 98–99, 102, 129–141; developing observation charts, 137–141; direct vs. indirect, 132–133; guidelines for documenting, 134–137; hidden observation, 133–134; joint observation, 132; less-structured vs. structured observation, 133; longitudinal observation, 130; nonparticipant observation, 131–132; observation in natural settings vs. controlled environments (field vs. lab), 134; open vs. hidden, 130; participant vs. nonparticipant observation, 131–132; projection, 136; repeated observations, 130; single vs. multiple observations, 130–131; stereotyping, 136; subjective interpretations, 136; third-party observation vs. self-observation, 130, 134; time stamps, 137; triggering factors, 137

target audience, 248–249

target population, 106–109

terminology, 238

testing, 99–100, 102, 155–158, 159, 227; 3-D visual representations, 161; case studies, 158; creative thinking and writing methods, 163; essays, 158; and evaluation, 210; fill-in-the-blank tests, 158; narrative methods, 162; open vs. closed tests, 156–157; oral tests, 157; photovoice, 161; practice exercises, 158; presentation, 161;

role-playing, 158; short-answer tests, 158; speech bubbles, 161; story dialogue, 162; storytelling, 162; testing strategies, 222–223; visual methods, 160–161. *See also* alternative methods for data collection

textual source, 216

texts, data analysis for, 188–193

third-party observation vs. self-observation, 134

timelines, 115

training materials, 245

transcribe, 101

transformation, of data, 177

transparency, 248

triangulation, 20–21, 32, 94–95, 104, 116, 143; of methods, 20–21; of researchers, 20–21; of sources, 20–21

trustworthy, 65

user-friendly interventions, 220

validity, 16–19, 96; guidelines in achieving validity and reliability, 20–23, 31, 32, 123, 155

valuation, 103

variable, 178–179; interval variable, 179; nominal variable, 179; ordinal variable, 179

video, 98

video log or vlog, 240

visualization, 102

visual testing methods, 102, 160–161

walk-through, 223

website, 240

weighted decision matrix, 220

willingness, 103

work plan / research plan, 92, 109–117

workshop, 239–240

zoom in and out, 78–79, **79**